Access to Medical Records and Reports
A Practical Guide

Robert Cowley

Barrister-at-Law, of Lincoln's Inn

Foreword by Dr Graham Burt
Editor, *Journal of the Medical Defence Union*

RADCLIFFE MEDICAL PRESS, OXFORD and NEW YORK

© 1994 Radcliffe Medical Press Ltd
15 Kings Meadow, Ferry Hinksey Road, Oxford OX2 0DP

Radcliffe Medical Press Inc
141 Fifth Avenue, Suite N, NY 10010, USA

British Library Cataloguing in Publication Data

A catalogue record for this book is available from the British Library

ISBN 1 870905 59 8

Typeset by Advance Typesetting Ltd, Oxfordshire
Printed and bound in Great Britain

Contents

Foreword

A request for access to information held by a doctor about his patient always raises doubts in the doctor's mind. I have a duty of confidentiality, but is it absolute? Is it overridden by a law or by a duty to society? Has the patient given consent and, if so, is the consent properly informed? Might I withhold information which I consider detrimental to the patient's interests?

Many doctors will speak to the Medical Defence Union when faced with these doubts. At the MDU, we receive more than 10 000 enquiries each year from GPs and their staff. Twenty-five per cent of these calls refer to disclosure of medical information, records or reports.

Robert Cowley has written an excellent guide in which he leads us through the relevant principles and legislation in an authoritative fashion. He clarifies the issues masterfully in a text which is highly readable. I commend this book to doctors, their staff and hospital managers, all of whom will benefit from its lucid review of access to medical records and reports.

DR GRAHAM BURT
Editor, *Journal of the Medical Defence Union*
August 1993

Preface

Never has there been a greater need for an accurate and reliable guide to the law governing access to medical records. The past decade has witnessed the introduction of three major pieces of legislation conferring on patients the right of access to their medical records: the Data Protection Act 1984; the Access to Medical Reports Act 1988; and the Access to Health Records Act 1990. This legislation, and the increasing awareness among patients of their legal rights, mean that healthcare providers need to understand the subject. This book, therefore, is an attempt to meet this need by providing hospital managers, doctors and other healthcare professionals with a clear, practical guide to the relevant law.

For easy reference, the book is divided into three sections: Patient Access; Access and Litigation; and Professional Confidence and Third Party Access. At the end of the book the principal legislation, regulations and health services guidance are reproduced.

Finally, I should like to acknowledge the debt I owe to Dr John Keown, Chris Vellenoweth, and the Department of Health, each of which, on reading the draft of the book, made many thought-provoking and constructive comments. I remain, of course, solely responsible for the accuracy of this book.

ROBERT COWLEY
August 1993

Patient Access

1

Access to Computerized Medical Records

Introduction

In January 1980 the Council of Europe published a convention which aimed to protect privacy in response to the expansion of information and communication technology. Under the convention party states would be able to refuse the sending of personal information to countries where there were no comparable safeguards. In May 1980 the convention was signed by the United Kingdom, and in 1984 the Data Protection Act was passed.

The Act, which is both lengthy and complex, places legal obligations on those described in the Act as 'data users', who record and use 'personal data'. They must register their use of personal data with the Data Protection Registry and comply with the Data Protection Principles. These statutory Principles require that the obtaining and processing of personal data be done fairly and lawfully. The Act also gives new rights to those about whom personal data is recorded, described in the Act as 'data subjects'. These include certain rights of access to the data, and a right to compensation for damage resulting from inaccuracies in the data. A data subject may also apply to court for an order to erase or amend inaccuracies in personal data which concern him.

Which records are covered by the Act?

The Act is only concerned with regulating the use of 'personal data' which is defined in section 1(3) as:

> . . . data consisting of information which relates to a living individual who can be identified from that information (or from other information in the possession of the data user), including any expression of opinion.

There are several qualifications to this definition, five of which need to be noted in the present context.

Firstly, in order for information to constitute 'data', and therefore 'personal data' it must be:

> . . . recorded in a form in which it can be processed automatically in response to instructions given for that purpose. (section 1(2))

Old medical records may be stored on microfilm, from which they can be extracted manually or by microprocessor. As data is defined as information which is processed automatically, only in the latter instance will the Act apply.

Secondly, any operation performed solely for the purpose of preparing the text of documents does not constitute 'processing' as defined by the Act (section 1(8)). This is intended to ensure that by using a simple word processor, with the sole purpose of producing a letter or report, a person does not fall within the regulatory framework provided by the Act, even though the letter or report may contain personal information concerning an individual.

Thirdly, the data must be processed by reference to the 'data subject', (section 1(2) as qualified by section 1(7). Processing which incidentally reveals personal data, such as information collated for audit purposes, will not fall within the scope of the Act.

Fourthly, information is only 'personal data' when it relates to a living individual. Once a patient has died, information about them is exempt from the provisions of the Act (section 1(3)).

Finally, statements of intent, but not statements of opinion, are expressly excluded from the definition of 'personal data' (section 1(3)). This might have presented an opportunity for avoiding patient scrutiny of sensitive data by disguising information as a statement of intention. However, in guidance issued by the Data Protection Registrar, he warns that:

> The Registrar expects this exclusion to apply only where the data user has a clear unsettled intention. He does not consider the exclusion can be used to disguise an opinion by phrasing it as an intention. The Registrar considers that both the way in which the information is recorded and the way in which it is used by the data user will be relevant in deciding this issue. (paragraph 3.4, Guideline 2, 'The Definitions')

For example, if a doctor were to enter a note into a patient's records which read 'At future consultations I intend to beware of this patient's hypochondria', the Data Protection Registrar may well take the view that the doctor in question is seeking to disguise a statement of opinion as a statement of intention in order to take it outside the scope of the Act and, thereby, prevent the patient gaining access to it.

Applications for access

Who may apply for access?

1 *The patient*
Under section 21(1) an individual is entitled:

(a) to be informed by any data user whether the data held by him include personal data of which the individual is the data subject; and

(b) to be supplied by any data user with a copy of the information constituting any such personal data held by him.

For children to exercise their right of access they must be able to understand the nature of the application. The age at which they are able to do this will depend on their maturity and intellect. It will be seen (on page 8) that before responding to an application for access, an appropriate health professional should be consulted to ensure, for example, that granting access is not likely to cause the patient serious harm. The assessment of whether a child has the requisite capacity to make a valid application should be made at this stage. In the majority of cases, if a child is sufficiently mature to consent to minor treatment then he or she will be capable of making a valid application for access. However, if it is unclear from a child's medical records whether he or she has the requisite capacity, the appropriate health professional will either need to interview the child or obtain a written declaration from a parent of the child confirming that the child understands the nature of the application (*see* HC (87)26, appendix 1, at para 2, as amended: reproduced on pages 120–1).

2 *A person acting on behalf of the patient*
Section 21 does not specify that someone acting on the patient's behalf can make an application for information. However, the Act appears to permit agents to make applications, as the 'non-disclosure' provisions preserving confidentiality do not apply to the patient or the patient's agents (section 34(6)). Whether the agent has a right to demand to be provided with access in accordance with section 21 is less clear. However, in guidance issued by the Data Protection Registrar, the view is taken that:

There is no reason why an intellectually capable individual should not make a subject access request through an agent. A data user who receives such a request should reply to it if he is satisfied that the individual has authorised the agent to make the request . . . [such as] written authority signed by the individual. (para 2.32, Guideline 5)

Failure to respond to such an application may therefore result in the Registrar serving on the health authority an enforcement notice (*see* 'Breach and enforcement', page 15).

3 *A person having parental responsibility for the child*

Although not specified by the Act, a person having parental responsibility for a child is entitled, in accordance with common-law principles, to apply for access to the child's records, provided that the application is in the child's interests. This person will normally be a parent of the child, but could also be, for example, a local authority or grandparent.

It appears that the parental right to make the application ceases once children can understand the nature of, and thus make applications themselves. As was stated by Lord Scarman in *Gillick v. West Norfolk and Wisbech Area Health Authority* [1985] 3 All ER 402 at 422:

> The parental right yields to the child's right to make his own decisions when he reaches a sufficient understanding and intelligence to be capable of making up his own mind on the matter requiring decision.

(This interpretation of the common law is consistent with the approach adopted by the Access to Health Records Act 1990.)

HC (87)26 (at appendix 1, para 2, as amended) advises that where an application is received by a parent seeking access to a child's medical records, a declaration should be obtained from the parent stating that the child does not understand the nature of the application (and thereby lacks the requisite consent to make the application). This declaration can then be accepted, unless there is evidence to the contrary, such as the child having previously made a successful application for access.

Where the child is capable of making an application, an application by a parent must be treated as an application by a person acting on the patient's behalf, rather than by a person exercising parental rights.

4 *A person acting on behalf of any individual who is incapable by reason of mental disorder of managing his or her own affairs*

By virtue of section 21(9), the Secretary of State may make regulations enabling a request for access to be made on behalf of any individual who is incapable by reason of mental disorder of managing his or her own affairs. Proposals for an order to be laid down under section 21(9) were circulated as long ago as August 1987, but no such order has yet been made. Whether any order will be made under the section remains to be seen.

To whom should the application be made?

An application for access must be made to the person who 'holds' the personal data to which the application relates, described in the Act as the 'data user' (section 21(2)). A person will be the holder of personal data if:

(a) the data form part of a collection of data processed or intended to be processed by or on behalf of that person . . .; and

(b) that person (either alone or jointly with other persons) controls the contents and use of the data comprised in the collection . . .

Control over the contents and use of the data is central to the concept of holding. The data user must contribute to control of both the content of the data and its use, although it is not necessary to process the data personally. In practice, decisions about the content and use of data will normally be made by individual employees. However, employees will not normally be data users themselves since they will be merely exercising control on behalf of the employer.

(c) the data in the form in which they have been or are intended to be processed as mentioned in paragraph (a) above or (though not for the time being in that form) in a form into which they have been converted after being so processed and with a view to being further so processed on a subsequent occasion. (section 1(5))

This third criterion is designed simply to cover data converted into another form after being processed, from which it is intended to process the data on some subsequent occasion. For example, data which is only processed occasionally may be processed on a disc but be stored on magnetic tape when not in use. Such data continue to be 'held', despite not being in the form in which they were processed. The purpose of the criterion is simply to plug what would otherwise be a loophole in the Act.

Hospitals do not in law ordinarily constitute 'persons' and cannot therefore be data users. However, NHS Trusts (established under section 5 of the National Health Service and Community Care Act 1990) and (by virtue of paragraph 8, Part III, Schedule 5, National Health Service Act 1977), regional and district health authorities are legal 'persons' and are therefore capable of holding data. Accordingly, an NHS Trust will hold data within its control, and district and regional health authorities will hold data controlled at district and regional level respectively. An application for access should therefore be addressed to the chief executive of the appropriate Trust hospital, regional or district health authority, and not the responsible consultant. It is quite possible for two 'persons', whether individuals or health service bodies, to hold the same data.

In the private health sector, the appropriate company controlling the contents and use of the data will be the data user to whom the application should be made. A partnership is not a legal person and therefore each partner will hold the data held by the partnership. Accordingly an application may be made to any member of the partnership. (Hereafter, reference to 'health service bodies' may be taken as also including reference to general practitioners).

The application

It is important to note that the right of access created by section 21(1) is not activated until three criteria are satisfied.

Firstly, the application must be made in writing (section 21(2)). In the absence of any indication to the contrary, a request under paragraph (a) of section 21 (ie a request to be informed whether the health service body holds any personal data concerning the patient) must be treated as also including a request under paragraph (b) of section 21 (ie a request to be supplied with that information). Similarly a request for information under both paragraphs (a) and (b) must be treated as one application (section 21(2)). However, where separate entries have been made in the Data Protection Register in respect of data held for different purposes, a separate application must be made in respect to each entry (section 21(3)). A health authority may, for example, make separate entries in respect of an employee's medical and employment records. In such a case, the employee seeking to gain access to both would have to make two separate requests: one in relation to employment records and another in relation to medical records.

Secondly, the applicant must provide the health service body with such information as it may reasonably require to identify the person making the request and to locate the information sought (section 21(4)(a)).

Thirdly, the Act permits a fee (currently £10) to be charged for processing the request. Where such a charge is made, the appropriate fee may be required in advance of access being granted (section 21(2)). However, it is important to note that, although access can be denied until the requisite payment is made, nonpayment does not justify delay in processing the application. The 40 day period within which an application must be processed (*see* page 10) runs from the date on which the first two criteria above are satisfied, irrespective of whether or not payment is received at that time (*see* HC (87)26 at para 3, page 118).

Dealing with applications for access

The duty to consult

Where the data are held not by a health professional but, for example, by a health service body, the holder must consult the 'appropriate health professional' before responding to a valid application for access (Data

Protection (Subject Access Modification) Order 1987 SI 1987/1903). This is to ensure that, for example, information is not disclosed which is likely to cause the patient serious harm (*see* Safeguards and exemptions, pages 10–11).

The term 'appropriate health professionals' is defined in paragraph 4(6) of the order as being:

(a) the medical practitioner or dental practitioner who is currently or was most recently responsible for the clinical care of the data subject in connection with the matters to which the information which is the subject of the request; or

(b) where there is more than one such practitioner, the practitioner who is the most suitable to advise on the matters to which the information which is the subject of the request relates; or

(c) where there is no practitioner available falling within sub-paragraph (a) or (b) above, a health professional who has the necessary experience and qualifications to advise on the matters to which the information which is the subject of the request relates.

Several medical practitioners will sometimes have been concurrently responsible for the clinical care of the applicant. In such a situation, it is for the chief executive of the responsible health service body to decide which is the most appropriate to advise on the application. The appointed practitioner (or in the absence of a practitioner, other health professional) should then consult other practitioners and health professionals who have had a significant input into the patient's care.

What information must be disclosed in response to an application for access?

The information to be supplied, in response to an application for access, is that held at the time when the request is received. There is an exception, where the data are amended or deleted between the time the request is received and the time the information is supplied, provided that the amendment or deletion would have been made regardless of the request (section 21(7)). Health service bodies are thus prevented from amending the data in order to cover up an inaccuracy and from erasing data they do not wish to be disclosed, but not from updating their records.

From a practical viewpoint, probably of most concern to health service bodies and general practitioners alike, is section 21(1), which provides:

Where any of the information . . . is expressed in terms which are not intelligible without explanation, the information shall be accompanied by an explanation of those terms.

How long does the health service body have in which to comply with a request for access?

Data users have 40 days in which to comply with the request. The period runs from the date on which the application is received (section 21(6)). However, where the authority is not supplied with the information that it needs to process the request, the 40 days run from the date on which it receives the requisite information (section 21(6)).

The Act places on data users certain obligations to preserve confidentiality. These ordinarily prevent data concerning, or provided by, an indentifiable third party from being disclosed without the third party's consent (*see* Safeguards and exemptions, below). The data user is not obliged to seek to obtain the requisite consent; he or she may instead simply choose to withhold such information. If, however, the data user chooses to seek third party consent to the disclosure, the 40 day period runs from the date on which the requisite consent is received or refused (section 21(6)).

Should a health service body wish to take advantage of the extension provisions, there is no requirement that it should seek to obtain the requisite information or consent within a specified period. However, any unreasonable delay on the part of the authority will constitute a breach of paragraph (a) of the Seventh Data Protection Principle, which requires that data subjects be given access without undue delay. Breach of this Principle, if notified to the Registrar, could lead to an enforcement notice being served on the body (*see* Breach and enforcement, page 15).

May a charge be made for allowing access?

Section 21(2) of the Act enables health service bodies to charge a fee (currently £10) for processing a request (The Data Protection (Subject Access) (Fees) Regulations 1987; SI 1987/1507). This applies irrespective of whether or not it holds any personal data concerning the applicant, or whether or not it is obliged to disclose the data. Although access may be withheld until the requisite payment is made, nonpayment does not excuse failure to process the request within the required 40 day period.

Safeguards and exemptions

There are numerous situations in which the right of access to personal data is excluded or has been modified, six of which are relevant in the present context.

1 *Health data*
On 9 November 1987, the Home Secretary, exercising his powers under section 29(1) of the Data Protection Act 1984, made the Data Protection

(Subject Access Modification) (Health) Order 1987 (SI 1987/1903). The Order applies to personal data concerning the physical or mental health of the data subject, provided that the data are either held by a health professional, or the information constituting the data was first recorded by, or on behalf of, a health professional (para 3).

The term 'health professional' is defined in Schedule 1 of the Order as follows:

> Registered medical practitioner, registered dentist, registered optician, registered pharmaceutical chemist or druggist, registered nurse, midwife, or health visitor, registered chiropodist, dietitian, occupational therapist, orthoptist or physiotherapist, clinical psychologist, child psychotherapist or speech therapist, art or music therapist employed by a health authority, health board or health and social services board, and scientists employed by such an authority or board as head of department.

The Order only permits access to be denied where disclosure would be likely to cause **serious harm** to the physical or mental health of the patient (para 4(2)(a)) or to reveal information either concerning, or provided by, an identifiable third party (other than where the individual concerned has either consented to the diclosure or is a health professional who has provided the information in a professional capacity) (para 4(2)(b) as qualified by para 4(3)(a)).

However, the order does not excuse health service bodies from supplying so much of the information as can be provided without causing serious harm to the patient or enabling the identity of a third party to be disclosed (or deduced), whether by omission of names, or other particulars, or otherwise (para 4(3)(b)).

2 Legal professional privilege

Any direct communications between lawyer and client (including communications between employers and salaried solicitors employed directly by them) enjoy privilege from disclosure, providing that the communications were made for the purpose of giving or receiving legal advise (section 31(2)). However, a report prepared by a third party, such as an accident report commissioned by a health authority and sent to its solicitor, will only enjoy privilege from disclosure where it was compiled in contemplation of litigation and that was the dominant purpose for which it was prepared (for information on the scope of legal professional privilege *see* page 38).

3 Statistics and research data

Personal data held for the purpose of preparing statistics or carrying out research are, by virtue of section 33(6), exempt from the subject access provisions, providing that the data are not used or disclosed for any other purpose. Furthermore, the results of the research must not be available in a form which identifies any of the data subjects. However, the exemption will not be lost where:

(a) the disclosure is to the data subject or a person acting on his behalf; or

(b) the data subject or any such person has requested or consented to the disclosure in question; or

(c) the disclosure is by a data user . . . to his servant or agent for the purpose of enabling the servant or agent to perform his functions as such; or

(d) the person making the disclosure has reasonable grounds for believing that the disclosure falls within any of the foregoing paragraphs. (section 34(6) as applied to section 33(6) by virtue of section 34(7))

4 *Prohibited disclosure*

The Secretary of State has the power under section 34(2) of the Act to exempt information from the access provisions, where disclosure of the information is prohibited or restricted by or under any other enactment. One such order has been made under the provision. The Order applies to adoption records and reports, and statements and records of the special education needs of children.

5 *Back-up data*

In certain cases, the data subject has a right to compensation for damage suffered as a result of the loss or impairment of personal data concerning him. Retaining 'back-up' copies of data is therefore good policy. Back-up copies are exempt from the subject access provisions, providing they are kept solely for the purpose of replacing other data if it is lost, destroyed, or impaired (section 34(4)). The exemption makes double access to the same information unnecessary. However, guidance issued by the Data Protection Registrar warns that if the data are kept so that they may be consulted whether or not the original files have been damaged, the exemption will be lost (*see* para C.6.3, Guideline 6, The Exemptions).

6 *Data incriminating the health service body*

The right against self-incrimination is a well-established principle of common law. The principle is preserved to an extent by section 34(9) which provides that:

A person [or here, health service body] need not comply with a notice, request or order under the subject access provisions if compliance would expose him to proceedings for any offence other than an offence under this Act.

Although not strictly a 'subject access exemption', its effect is the same.

Must the applicant be informed that information is being withheld on the basis of one of the exemptions?

Guideline 6, issued by the Registrar, advises that the data user need not inform the applicant that information is being withheld under one of these exemptions. If all the personal data concerning the applicant are exempt from disclosure, the health service body could properly reply 'We do not hold any personal data which we are required to reveal to you' (*see* para C.1.2).

Compensation for inaccuracy

If a patient suffers damage as the result of inaccurate data held by a health service body, for example where the inaccuracy causes the patient to receive inappropriate treatment, he or she is entitled to compensation for the harm and distress suffered (section 22(1)). However, the provision is of limited application. The right to compensation does not extend to persons who are not individuals (such as registered companies), or to other individuals who are not themselves the subject of the inaccurate data. Furthermore, for there to be compensation for distress, the inaccuracy must have caused the patient to suffer damage. 'Damage' is not defined in the Act and therefore must be given its natural meaning. In the Registrar's view, damage includes financial loss and physical harm, but does not include distress suffered by the individual (*see* para 3.3, Guideline 5, Individual Rights).

For the purposes of the section, data are defined as 'inaccurate' if they are incorrect or misleading as to any matter of fact (section 22(4)). A mere opinion, which does not purport to be a statement of fact, cannot be the subject of an action for compensation, even though an individual may dispute the opinion recorded about him. However, a statement of opinion may also contain an implied statement of fact. In *Smith v Land and Housing Corporation* (1884) 28 ChD 7, the vendor of a property described the tenant as being 'most desirable', when in actual fact he was in arrears with his rent. It was held that the description was not a mere opinion, but contained an implied assertion that nothing had occurred which could be regarded as rendering the tenant undesirable, thus enabling the purchaser to bring an action for misrepresentation. In view of the difficulties in distinguishing between statements of opinion and statements containing an implied assertion of fact, it is wise to avoid including speculative and unsubstantiated remarks in patients' records.

The right to compensation is subject to a further important qualification. There is no right to compensation where the data accurately record information received or obtained either from the patient, or from a third party, provided that:

(a) it is apparent that the information was so received whenever extracted from the data; and

(b) if the data subject has notified the data user that he regards the information as incorrect or misleading, again this must be apparent whenever the information is extracted from the data. (section 22(2))

Finally, a health service body also has a statutory defence against a claim for compensation, if it can show that it has taken such care as was reasonably required in the circumstances to ensure the accuracy of the data at the material time (section 22(3)). Whether reasonable steps were taken to ensure the accuracy of the data is a question of fact that has to be determined in each case. Factors such as the likelihood of damage, the cost of taking additional steps to ensure its accuracy, and standard practice in the health service will be relevant.

Rectification and erasure of inaccurate data

Where a health service body holds inaccurate data concerning a patient, the patient may apply to court for the rectification or erasure of the inaccurate data. The right is accorded by section 24 of the Act, which reflects the Fifth and Seventh Data Protection Principles. Section 24(1) provides that:

If a Court is satisfied on the application of a data subject that personal data held by a data user of which the applicant is the subject are inaccurate . . . [ie incorrect or misleading as to any matter of fact] the court may order the rectification or erasure of the data and of any data held by the data user and containing an expression of opinion which appears to the Court to be based on the inaccurate data.

Where the data accurately record information received or obtained by a health service body, whether from the patient or a third party, the Court may, instead of making an order that the data be amended or erased, make an order requiring the data to be supplemented by a statement of the true facts relating to the matters dealt with by the data (section 24(2)(a)). If the requirements of section 22(2) (*see* above) have not been complied with, the court may also make such an order as it thinks fit for securing compliance with those requirements (section 24(2)(b)).

The Court's discretion to order erasure is much more limited than its discretion to order rectification. The power to order erasure may be invoked only when two strict criteria are satisfied.

1 Either the patient must have suffered damage by reason of the inaccuracy, or access to the data must have been improperly obtained in circumstances giving entitlement to compensation.

2 There must be a substantial risk of further unauthorized disclosure of, or access to, the data in question (section 24(3)).

Breach and enforcement

An applicant refused access to his or her records in contravention of the Act is not entitled to compensation. However, an aggrieved patient may be able to obtain redress in one of two ways.

1 He or she may apply either to the County or High Court for an order requiring the health service body to comply with its obligations under the Act. However, a court is unable to grant an order if it considers that it would, under the circumstances, be unreasonable to do so, perhaps because of the frequency with which the applicant has made requests to the data user, or for some other reason (section 21(8)).

2 He or she may inform the Data Protection Registrar that the health service body has failed to comply with the Seventh Data Protection Principle. The Data Protection Registrar may then serve an enforcement notice on the body requiring it to grant access to the applicant (section 10(1)). The Registrar will usually try to resolve the dispute informally without serving a notice. If this is not possible, he will normally write to the chief executive of the body concerned, informing him that he is considering an enforcement notice and inviting representations as to why the notice should not be served. Having considered any representations, the Registrar will decide whether to serve the notice. Failure to comply with an enforcement notice is a criminal offence (section 10(9)), punishable by a potentially unlimited fine (section 19(2)). However, the health service body has a statutory defence to the charge if it can show that it used all due diligence to comply with the notice (section 10(9)).

2

Access to Non-Computerized Medical Records

Introduction

Until 1987, when the relevant part of the Data Protection Act 1984 came into force, patients had no general right of access to their medical records. The Act gave patients certain rights of access only to computerized medical records, thus creating an anomaly between computerized records and non-computerized records. The Access to Health Records Act 1990 was introduced to resolve this anomaly by granting patients similar rights of access to their manually held medical records.

Which records are covered by the Act?

The Act applies only to 'health records' which are defined in section 1(1)(a) as records which:

> . . . consist of information relating to the physical or mental health of an individual who can be identified from that information, or from that and other information in the possession of the holder of the record.

However, there are three important limitations to the scope of the Act.

1 The Act only applies to those records compiled after 1 November 1991, (other than to the extent that access to an earlier record is necessary to make intelligible any part of the record to which the applicant is entitled to have access) (section 5(1)(b)). This means that, although the Act did not come into force until 1 November 1991, notes made during an earlier period of treatment may still be subject to patient scrutiny.

2 The record must have been made:

> . . . by or on behalf of a *health professional* in connection with the *care* of the individual. (section 1(1)(b))

Who, for the purposes of the Act, is a 'health professional'?

Section 2 defines a 'health professional' as follows:

(a) a registered medical practitioner [including a person who is provisionally registered under section 15 or 21 of the Medical Act 1983 and is engaged in such employment as is mentioned in subsection (3) of that section];

(b) a registered dentist;

(c) a registered optician;

(d) a registered pharmaceutical chemist;

(e) a registered nurse, midwife or health visitor;

(f) a registered chiropodist, dietitian, occupational therapist, orthoptist or physiotherapist;

(g) a clinical psychologist, child psychotherapist or speech therapist;

(h) an art or music therapist employed by a health service body; and

(i) a scientist employed by such a body as head of department.

What is meant by 'care'?

'Care' is defined in section 11 of the Act as including:

. . . examination, investigation, diagnosis and treatment.

It is important to note that the definition does not require that the examination, investigation or diagnosis be made for the purposes of, or in connection with, treatment. This means that a patient may be able to obtain access to a report written by an independent doctor engaged, for example, by an employer or insurer.

3 The third limitation on the scope of the Act is that the definition of 'health record' provided by section 1:

. . . does not include any record which consists of information which the individual is, or but for any exemption would be, entitled to be supplied with a copy under section 21 of the Data Protection Act 1984 (right of access to personal data). (ie computerized records, *see* Chapter 1)

This is simply intended to avoid any overlap with the Data Protection Act 1984.

Applications for access

Who may apply for access?

1 *The patient* (section 3(1)(a))
Where the applicant is a child (ie under the age of 16 (section 11)), he or
she must, in the opinion of the record holder, be 'capable of understanding
the nature of the application' (section 4(1)). The age at which a child will
be capable of understanding the nature of the application will depend upon
the maturity and intellect of the child in question.

2 *Any person authorized in writing to do so on the patient's behalf* (section
3(1)(b))

3 *Where the patient is under 16, a person having parental responsibility for
the child* (section 3(1)(c))
A person having parental responsibility for the child will only have a right
of access to the child's records where, in the opinion of the holder:

• the child has consented to the application; or
• the child is incapable of understanding the nature of the application, and
  permitting access would be in the child's best interests (section 4(2)).

4 *Where the patient is incapable of managing his or her own affairs, any
person appointed by a court to manage those affairs* (section 3(1)(e))

5 *Where the patient has died, the patient's personal representative and any
person who may have a claim arising out of the death* (section 3(1)(f))
The right of access conferred on both the deceased's personal representative
and any person who may have a claim arising out of the patient's death must
be read in conjunction with section 5(4), which states that:

> . . . access shall not be given . . . to any part of the record which, in the
> opinion of the holder of the record, would disclose information which is
> not relevant to any claim which may arise out of the patient's death.

Nor may access be permitted to the deceased's record if it includes a note,
made at his or her request, that he or she did not wish access to be given
on such an application (section 4(3)).
   The principal effect of the section is to enable the deceased's administrator
or executor to obtain evidence which may be needed to bring an action on
behalf of the deceased's dependants under the Fatal Accidents Act 1976 (as
amended). This provides that:

> If death is caused by any wrongful act, neglect or default which is such
> as would (if death had not ensued) have entitled the person injured to

maintain an action and recover damages in respect thereof, the person who would have been liable if death had not ensued shall be liable to an action for damages, notwithstanding the death of the person injured. (section 1(1))

The Fatal Accidents Act 1976 provides for recovery in respect of two types of loss.

1 In respect of a death occurring after 1982, the spouse of the deceased, or the parents of a minor who never married, may claim a fixed sum of £7500 for bereavement.

2 A 'dependent' may claim for the loss of financial support provided by the deceased. For the purposes of such a claim the following are regarded as dependants:

- the spouse or former spouse of the deceased, or the person who was living as the spouse of the deceased in the same household immediately before the date of the death, and had been so living for at least two years
- any parent or other descendant of the deceased, or person treated by the deceased as his parent
- any child or other descendant of the deceased, or any person who has been treated by the deceased as a child of the family in relation to any marriage of the deceased, and
- any person who is, or is the issue of, a brother, sister, uncle or aunt of the deceased.

An action under the Fatal Accidents Act 1976 is normally taken on behalf of the dependants by the executor or administrator of the deceased. However, where there is no personal representative, or if no action is brought within six months, any dependant who is entitled to benefit under the Act may sue in his or her own name on behalf of himself and the others. (Reference should be made to other sources for a fuller explanation of the Fatal Accidents Act 1976.[1])

To whom should the application be made?

The application must be made to the 'holder' of the record to which access is sought. The 'holder' is defined as follows:

(a) in the case of a record made by, or by a health professional employed by, a general practitioner:
  (i) the patient's general practitioner, that is to say, the general practitioner on whose list the patient is included; or

---

[1] See *Winfeld and Jolowicz on Tort* (13th edn), 1989, Sweet & Maxwell.

(ii) where the patient has no general practitioner, the [family health services authority] . . . on whose medical list the patient's most recent general practitioner was included;

(b) in the case of a record made by a health professional for purposes connected with the provision of health services by a health service body: the health service body by which or on whose behalf the record is held;

(c) in any other case, the health professional by whom or on whose behalf the record if held. (section 1(2))

'Health service body' as mentioned above in (b) is in turn defined in section 11 as a health authority (within the meaning of the National Health Service Act 1977); or a National Health Service Trust (established under section 5 of the National Health Service and Community Care Act 1990).

The application

Any application must be made in writing (section 11) and must contain sufficient information to identify the patient. Where the application is made other than by the patient, the applicant must also establish that he or she is entitled to make the application (section 3(6)).

Dealing with applications for access

The duty to consult

Where the records to which access is being sought are held by either a health service body or health services authority, the holder of the records is under an obligation to take advice from 'the appropriate health professional' when deciding how to respond to the application for access (section 8(1)).

In the case of the record being held by a health services body (ie an NHS Trust or health authority), the 'appropriate health professional' is defined as follows:

(a) where . . . one or more medical or dental practitioners are currently responsible for the clinical care of the patient, that practitioner or, as the case may be, such one of those practitioners as is most suitable to advise the body on the matter in question;

(b) where paragraph (a) above does not apply but one or more medical or dental practitioners are available who, for the purposes connected with the provisions of such services by the body, have been responsible for the clinical care of the patient, that practitioner or, as the case may be, such one of those practitioners as was most recently so responsible; and

(c) where neither paragraph (a) nor paragraph (b) above applies, a health professional who has the necessary experience and qualifications to advise the body on the matter in question. (section 7(2))

Several medical practitioners will sometimes have been concurrently responsible for the clinical care of the applicant. In such a situation, it is for the chief executive of the health service body responsible to decide which is the most appropriate to advise on the application. The appointed practitioner (or in the absence of a practitioner, other health professional) should then consult other practitioners and health professionals who have had significant input into the patient's care.

In the case of the record being held by a health services authority, the 'appropriate health professional' is defined as follows:

(a) where the patient's most recent general practitioner is available, that practitioner; and

(b) where that practitioner is not available, a registered medical practitioner who has the necessary experience and qualifications to advise the . . . [authority] on the matter in question. (section 7(3))

How long does the holder have in order to comply with a request for access?

Requests for access need to be dealt with promptly. Where the application relates to a record, or part of a record, which was made during the 40 days immediately preceding the date of the application, access must be given within 21 days of the application (section 3(5)(a)). In any other case, access must be given within 40 days of the date of the application (section 3(5)(b)). The 'date of the application' is not defined in the Act, but a court would almost certainly rule this to be the day on which the application is received rather than any earlier point in time, such as the date on the application itself, or the date on which it was posted. Any other interpretation could, if the application was significantly delayed, result in the holder of the record unwittingly being in breach of the Act.

May a charge be made for allowing access?

Dealing with applications for access may prove to be time consuming and expensive. However, no charge may be made for granting access except:

• where access is given to information, none of which was recorded during the 40 days immediately preceding the application: in which case a fee not exceeding the maximum prescribed under section 21 of the Data Protection Act 1984 may be charged (section 3(4)(a)) (currently £10); or

- where a copy of a record or extract is supplied to the applicant: in which case a fee not exceeding the cost of making the copy and (where applicable) the cost of posting it to him may be charged (section 3(4)(b)).

Safeguards and exemptions

The Act recognizes that there are circumstances in which information should be withheld. Access must not be given to any part of a patient's notes that would disclose information which in the opinion of the holder:

- would be likely to cause **serious harm** to the physical or mental health of the patient or of any other individual
- relates to, or has been provided by, an identifiable third party, unless the third party either consents to the disclosure, or is a health professional who has provided the information in a professional capacity (section 5(1)(a) as qualified by section 5(2)).

Where the application is by someone other than the patient or a person authorized to make the application on his behalf, a further safeguard will apply:

- the holder must not disclose information which he or she believes was provided by the patient in the expectation that it would not be disclosed to the applicant, or obtained as a result of any examination or investigation to which the patient consented in the expectation that the information would not be disclosed (section 5(3)).

Where the applicant is entitled to access the whole of the record he or she must be permitted access to the actual record itself (section 3(2)(a)). Where the applicant's right of access is limited to a certain part of the record, the Act states that the applicant should be given access to an 'extract' setting out the relevant part (section 3(2)(b)). The Act does not define the term 'extract' but it would appear that the term enables the holder of the record to give the applicant access to the relevant part of the actual record itself, or should the applicant prefer, to a copy of the relevant part. In either case, the applicant must be provided with a copy of the record or extract (section 3(2)(c)). He or she must also be provided with an explanation of any terms contained in the record which would otherwise be unintelligible (section 3(3)).

Correction of inaccurate health records

Where the applicant considers that any information to which he or she has been given access is incorrect, misleading or incomplete, a request may be made in writing that the record be corrected (section 6(1)). On receiving a request for correction, the holder of the record shall:

(a) if he is satisfied that the information is inaccurate, make the necessary correction

(b) if he is not so satisfied, make in the part of the record in which the information is contained a note of the matters in respect of which the information is considered by the applicant to be inaccurate; and

(c) in either case, without requiring a fee, supply the applicant with a copy of the correction or note. (section 6(2))

Disputes and enforcement

The Secretary of State has the power to require the holders of health records to make arrangements for dealing with any complaints that they have failed to comply with the requirements of the Act. Once the (as yet unspecified) complaints procedure (if any) has been exhausted, compliance with the Act may be enforced by the courts under section 8(1), which provides that:

. . . where the court is satisfied, on an application made by the person concerned within such period as may be prescribed by the rules of the court, that the holder of a health record has failed to comply with any requirement of this Act, the court may order the holder to comply with that requirement.

Criminal liability

The Act does not provide any sanction for its breach. Whether or not failure to comply with a given statute involves commission of the common law offence of disobeying a statute, depends upon the construction of the statute in question. Traditionally, there has been a presumption that where the statute 'prohibits a matter of public grievance to the liberties and securities of the subject . . . all acts or omissions contrary to the prohibition or command of the statute are misdemeanours at common law, punishable on indictment'.[2] However, in R. v. Horseferry Road Justices, Ex parte Independent Broadcasting Corporation [1986] 1 WLR 132, the Divisional Court took the view that, in relation to modern statutes, the presumption, if any, is the other way. Therefore clear language, or a very clear inference, is required for the offence to apply. Furthermore, where the Act provides

[2]Archbold, *Criminal pleading evidence and practice*, (Vol. 1, para. 1–6), (44th edn), 1991, Sweet & Maxwell.

some mechanism for enforcement, such as section 8, this presumption will be particularly difficult to rebut. As no such clear language or inference is contained within the Access to Health Records Act 1990, it is unlikely that criminal liability would be incurred for failing to comply with the Act.

Civil liability

A person who is harmed by another's failure to comply with a statute will be able to recover damages where the statute so intends. In practice, it can be difficult to determine precisely what the intention or purpose of a statute is.

It has been said that where an Act creates an obligation, and enforces its performance in a specified manner (in the case of the Access to Health Records Act 1990, by an application to court), then, as a general rule, that performance cannot be enforced in any other manner (*Doe d. Murray v. Bridges* (1831) 1 B & Ad 847). The authorities are, however, by no means consistent. Moreover, the vast majority of cases in which the courts have followed this general rule have been concerned with the liability of public bodies to the general public. Where the duty is owed to a limited and ascertainable class of individuals, as in the present context, the courts have seemed more willing to award damages, despite the availability of alternative means of enforcement. Whether failure to provide an applicant with access to a health record in accordance with the provisions of the Act results in civil liability to the applicant is, therefore, unclear. Even where the courts rule that an applicant who has wrongly been denied access is entitled to damages, any award would usually be nominal, the applicant having suffered no harm.

3

Access to Medical Reports

Introduction

On 1 January 1989 the Access to Medical Reports Act 1988 came into force, representing a further step in the general trend towards greater patient access to their medical records. The Act gives patients the right to see certain medical reports written about them for the use of third parties. However, the Act has a much more limited application than its short title suggests. In the words of the Act's sponsor, Archie Kirkwood MP, 'It is a finely focused and modest measure'.

Which reports are covered by the Act?

The scope of the Act is restricted in two ways.

Firstly, the Act only applies to the narrow category of medical reports compiled for 'employment purposes or insurance purposes' (section 1). The explanation for this is to be found in the background to the Act. Prior to the Bill's first reading, progress had been made in talks, between the medical profession and the Department of Health, aimed at agreeing a voluntary code of practice which would facilitate greater access to those medical records not stored in 'computerized' form and therefore falling outside the provisions of the Data Protection Act 1984. (The code of practice, 'Communicating Information to Patients and Their Own Medical Records', was never in fact issued and access to manually held records is now dealt with by the Access to Health Records Act 1990.) There remained, however, a gap in relation to medical reports compiled for 'external consumption'. The Act was intended solely to fill this gap but in limiting the scope of the Act to those reports compiled for insurance or employment purposes, the Act only partially does so.

The definition of 'employment purposes or insurance purposes' in section 2(1) is crucial in determining whether the provisions of the Act apply to any given case.

Employment purposes

'Employment purposes' are defined as:

> the purposes in relation to the individual of any person by whom he is or has been, or is seeking to be, employed (whether under a contract of service or otherwise). (section 2(1))

In order for a report to qualify as being for employment purposes it must, therefore, be compiled for the use of a past, present or prospective employer. Reports of occupational health physicians concerning employees' fitness to work will therefore be regarded as having been compiled for 'employment purposes' (but *see* Clinical care, page 27). However, the fact that the report may have a bearing on the patient's employment is not in itself sufficient to bring the report within the ambit of the Act. For example, a practitioner who is requested by the Department of Transport Medical Advisory Branch to provide a medical report in support of a heavy goods vehicle licence application need not comply with the provisions of the Act, although he must still obtain the patient's consent before disclosing confidential information.

Insurance purposes

The Act takes a similar approach in relation to the definition of 'insurance purposes' which are defined as:

> . . . the purposes in relation to the individual of any person carrying on an insurance business with whom the individual has entered into, or is seeking to enter into, a contract of insurance, and 'insurance business' and 'contract of insurance' have the same meaning as in the Insurance Companies Act 1982. (section 2(1))

Although a detailed analysis of the Insurance Companies Act 1982 is outside the scope of this book, it is particularly important to note that in order for a report to fall within the scope of the Act, the patient must either have entered into a contract of insurance with the applicant or be seeking to do so. Consequently, a report prepared for the Motor Insurers' Bureau will not be seen to be for insurance purposes as defined in the Act. Neither will reports requested by the Department of Social Security Divisional Medical Officer relating to a patient's claim for sickness or invalidity benefit.

The second major restriction on the scope of the Act is that the report must have been supplied by a registered medical practitioner who is, or has been, responsible for the 'clinical care' of the person about whom the report is concerned (section 2(1)).

Clinical care

'Care' is defined in section 2(1) as including:

> . . . examination, investigation or diagnosis for the purposes of, or in connection with, any form of medical treatment.

This deliberately excludes reports based upon an examination by an independent medical practitioner who is not subject to the same doctor-patient relationship. The doctor who has been acting exclusively to further the patient's health will have had access to confidential information given on the basis of that relationship. However, on preparing a report for an employer or insurer, the doctor must assume a duty to that third party; this not only alters the nature of the doctor-patient relationship but also creates a potential conflict of interest.

In the vast majority of cases, it will be obvious whether or not the medical practitioner is, or has been, responsible for the clinical care of the individual about whom the report concerns. Particular problems arise, however, in relation to occupational health physicians, whether employed in the NHS or the private sector.

An examination made for the purposes of statutory screening, in accordance with the Health and Safety at Work Act 1974, or in order to provide simple advice to employees as to their fitness to continue in employment, is not made for the purpose of, or in connection with, medical treatment. However, where the physician's duties extend beyond this, to providing first-aid in the event of an accident at work, for example, the legal position is less clear. Until the courts provide more detailed criteria for determining whether or not a medical practitioner is responsible for the clinical care of an individual, in circumstances where an occupational physician's duties include, for example, providing first-aid, it should be assumed that the Act does apply. If the doctor is pressured by the employer to provide a medical report concerning an employee, without complying with the Act, an application can be made to the County Court for a ruling (section 8).

It is important to note that the scope of the Access to Health Records Act 1990 (see Chapter 2) is not limited to medical records, but may also include medical reports. Nor does the 1990 Act require that the record or report be written by a medical practitioner who is responsible for the patient's treatment. Accordingly, by utilizing the Access to Health Records Act 1990, a patient may be able to gain access to a medical report written by an independent doctor, despite being unable to do so under the Access to Medical Reports Act 1988.

Requests for medical reports

No person may apply to a medical practitioner for a report about a patient without first obtaining the patient's written consent (section 3(1)). The Act also requires the potential applicant to inform the patient in writing of his or her rights under the Act when seeking the requisite consent (section 3(2)). If the patient consents to the application proceeding, he or she may inform the applicant that he or she wishes to have access to the report. The applicant must then both inform the doctor that this is so when requesting the report, and at the same time, notify the patient that he or she has requested the report (section 4(1)).

Dealing with requests for medical reports

Patient access to the report

Where the patient has informed the applicant that he or she wishes to be given access to the report, the doctor may not then release the report unless either the patient has first been given access to the report, or:

> the period of 21 days beginning with the date of the making of the application has elapsed without his having received any communication from the patient concerning arrangements for the individual to have access to it. (section 4(2))

From what date is the period of 21 days calculated?
The use of the words 'beginning with' makes it clear that the day on which the application is made is to be included when calculating the period of 21 days (*Hare v. Gocher* [1962] 2 QB 641). Unfortunately, however, the Act provides no assistance in determining 'the date of the making of the application'. This could be one of at least three points in time: the date specified on the application itself; the date of posting the application; or the date on which the application is received at the practitioner's surgery or other place of work. Until the courts clarify this point, practitioners are advised to calculate the period of 21 days from the date on which the application is received.

Does the Act provide for a change of mind by the patient?
Should a patient inform the applicant that he or she does not wish to be given access to the report, the Act does cater for a subsequent change of mind, provided the patient notifies the practitioner in writing before the report is supplied (section 4(3)(b)). The practitioner is then prevented from releasing the report until either the patient has been given access to it, or

21 days have elapsed (from the date of the notification of the change of mind, rather than from the date of the application) and no communication has been received from the patient concerning arrangements for access.

The Act states that any notification required or authorized under the Act can be given by post (section 9(b)). Section 7 of the Interpretation Act 1978 provides that where a statute authorizes any document to be served or sent by post, unless the contrary intention appears, the service is deemed to take place at the time at which the letter would be delivered in the ordinary course of post (provided that the letter is properly stamped and addressed). Therefore, as a matter of law, if the notification is posted on 1 March, for example, but is not received by the practitioner until 1 April, he or she may then supply the report to the applicant without further delay. As a matter of practice, however, it is simpler and safer to calculate the period of 21 days from the date on which the notification is received.

Must the patient be given access to the actual report itself?

Section 6(3) permits the practitioner to choose whether to permit the patient access to the actual report itself or to supply a copy of the report.

Safeguards and exemptions

The Department of Health has consistently taken the view that there should be common criteria for disclosure in the limited field of medical records. The Act, therefore, contains exemptions parallel to those contained in the Data Protection Act 1984 (as amended by the Data Protection (Subject Access Modification) (Health) Order 1987: SI 1987/1903). It is important to note at the outset that the exemptions contained in the Act enable only the relevant part or parts of the report to be withheld from the patient.

- A doctor is not obliged to disclose, and should not disclose, any part of the report which he or she believes would be 'likely to cause **serious harm** to the physical or mental health of the patient or others' (section 7(1)).
- Nor is the doctor obliged to do so if disclosure would reveal either information about another individual, or the identity of another person who has supplied information about the patient. This exemption does not apply if the person concerned either consents to the patient having access to the information, or is a 'health professional' who has provided the information in a professional capacity (section 7(2)). By virtue of section 2(1) the term 'health professional' has the same meaning as in the Data Protection (Subject Access Modification) (Health) Order 1987 (*see* page 11).
- Finally, in common with the Data Protection Act 1984, information which indicates the doctor's intentions in respect of the patient is also exempt from the provisions of the Act (section 7(1)).

Should the practitioner seek to rely on any of the exemptions in order to withhold disclosure, he or she must notify the patient in writing of the intention to do so (section 7(3)(a)). The practitioner is then prevented from releasing the report without written authorization from the patient (section 7(4)(b)).

May a charge be made for granting access to the report?

No change may be made for making a copy of the report available for the patient's inspection. However, where the patient is provided with a copy of the report, either at his or her request or with his or her consent, a reasonable fee may be charged to cover the cost of supplying it (section 4(4)).

Correction of inaccurate reports

Where the patient chooses to use the right of access, he or she may request in writing that the report be amended to the extent that it is considered to be inaccurate or misleading (section 5(2)). This does not amount to a right to demand amendments; whether or not the practitioner amends the report is a matter for professional judgement. If the practitioner is not prepared to accede to the patient's request, a statement must be attached to the report of the patient's views on the parts that have not been amended (section 5(2)(b)). Ultimately, however, if the report is wholly unsatisfactory to the patient, he or she may simply withdraw consent. Without the patient's consent, the report cannot be supplied to the applicant (section 5(3)). Finally, the patient has a right of access to the report during the six months after the report has been supplied to the applicant (section 6(2)).

Administrative requirements

Compliance with the Act requires an efficient system of administration. All correspondence should be date-stamped on its receipt.

The Act also requires the practitioner to retain a copy, 'for at least six months from the date on which it was supplied' (section 6(1)). The words 'at least' make it clear that the period of retention is to be exclusive of the date on which the report is supplied (*Rightside Properties Ltd v. Gray* [1975] Ch. 72).

Where the report is supplied by post, section 7 of the Interpretation Act 1978 (*see* page 29) will apply. The date of supplying the report will be the date on which the report would arrive at its destination in the ordinary course of post. It is therefore advisable to retain a copy of the report for at least six months from one week after the date of posting.

Disputes and enforcement

The principal means of enforcement is provided by section 8 which states that:

> If a court is satisfied on the application of an individual that any person, in connection with a medical report relating to that individual, has failed or is likely to fail to comply with any requirement of this Act, the Court may order that person to comply with that requirement.

As to criminal or civil liability for failure to comply with the provisions of the Act, *see* Chapter 2: Disputes and enforcement, page 23.

Access and Litigation

Introduction

Patients bringing personal injury claims will at some stage usually require access to their medical records, to determine either liability, for example where the claim is for medical negligence, or quantum (the amount of damages that may be obtained). To this end, the 'Rules of Court' provide for the 'discovery' of medical records. These rules differ, depending upon whether legal proceedings have been formally started by the issue of a writ or summons, or whether legal proceedings are merely proposed. Chapter 4 deals with access to medical records prior to the commencement of proceedings and Chapter 5 with access once proceedings have actually begun.

It will also be usual for the plaintiff to have to undergo at least two medical examinations, one by a doctor appointed by the plaintiff and one by a doctor appointed by the defendant, each of whom will prepare a report for their respectives sides. Each side will then wish to gain access to the other's report. This will prevent either party from conducting their case in ignorance of the strength of the other's, which in turn promotes an early settlement or, should the case proceed to trial, enables the issues to be defined in advance, thus saving time and expense. The disclosure of such reports is dealt with in Chapter 6.

4

Access with a View to Legal Proceedings

Introduction

Patients involved in personal injury litigation will at some stage seek access to their medical records. Where the claim arises out of a road accident or an accident at work, access will usually only be required after the commencement of legal proceedings (ie the issue of a writ). However, where an injury is sustained during medical treatment, it will often be difficult, if not impossible, to determine whether there is any basis for bringing a claim without first obtaining access to the relevant medication notes. Yet until 1971, patients' legal and medical advisers were required to do just that, disclosure of the notes normally being ordered only at the trial itself.

Section 31 of the Administration of Justice Act 1970 introduced the process known as 'pre-action discovery' whereby the High Court could order that a patient suspecting medical negligence should be given access to his or her notes so that he or she could receive informed legal advice without having to incur the expense of commencing formal proceedings (although in practice the application for access will be made by the patient's solicitor). The power to order pre-action discovery is now contained in section 33(2) of the Supreme Court Act 1981, which provides:

> On the application, in accordance with the rules of Court, of a person who appears to the Court to be likely to be a party to subsequent proceedings in that Court in which a claim in respect of personal injuries to a person, or in respect of a person's death, is likely to be made, the High Court shall, in such circumstances specified in the rules, have the power to order a person who appears to the Court to be likely to be a party to the proceedings and to be likely to have in his possession, custody or power any documents which are relevant to an issue arising or likely to arise out of that claim:
>
> (a) to disclose whether those documents are in his possession, custody or power; and
>
> (b) to produce such of those documents as are in his possession, custody or power to the applicant, or on such conditions as may be specified in the order.

In respect of claims where damages are likely to be less than £50 000 and are therefore brought to the County Court, the County Court has the same powers as the High Court to order pre-action discovery (section 52, County Courts Act 1984).

As we have seen, patients already enjoy a general right of access to their computerized medical records under the Data Protection Act 1984 and to their manually-held notes under the Access to Health Records Act 1990. However, it is doubtful whether either of the Acts has any significant effect on the use of pre-action discovery.

1 The Access to Health Records Act 1990 only applies to those records compiled after 1 November 1991, and as such will clearly be inappropriate in cases where the treatment under scrutiny was administered prior to this.

2 The obligation to provide a patient with access to his or her notes under the Access to Health Records Act 1990 may, in certain circumstances, be discharged by providing the patient with a copy of the notes. Although a solicitor may initially be contended with copies, he should at some stage require access to the originals in order to ensure that the copies received are complete; that no part of the documents, such as marginal notes, have failed to copy; and to ensure that the notes have not been added to at a later date (the use of a different pen may be obvious on the actual notes but impossible to detect on a photocopy).

3 Both the Data Protection Act 1984 and the Access to Health Records Act 1990, contain various exemptions. These permit information to be withheld if, for example, disclosure could cause the patient serious harm. No such exemptions apply to pre-action discovery, although the Court may, if appropriate, limit disclosure to the patient's legal and medical advisers.

4 Pre-action discovery is not limited to the patient's notes. An application may be made under section 33(2) for the disclosure of accident reports, or even the notes of other patients.

Far from becoming obsolete, as the number of medical negligence claims continues to rise, pre-action discovery will continue to become increasingly important. A detailed knowledge of pre-action discovery is therefore essential to anyone likely to be concerned with medical negligence litigation.

Which records are covered by the section?

The section refers to 'any documents which are relevant to an issue arising or likely to arise out of the claim'. Potentially, all medical, nursing, anaesthetic and surgical notes; laboratory test reports; X-ray films; consent forms;

clinical and other correspondence; and accident reports may be subject to pre-action discovery. This includes 'computerized' documents as well as manually-held documents (*see Derby & Co Ltd v. Weldon (No. 9)* [1991] 2 All ER 901).

However, there are two important limitations on the court's power to order disclosure.

1 The court is not empowered to order the disclosure of documents which would enjoy privilege from disclosure, had proceedings actually commenced. This is specifically enacted by Order 24, rule 7A(6) of the Rules of the Supreme Court 1965 (as amended) (hereafter RSC 1965), which states:

> No person shall be compelled by virtue of such an order to produce any documents which he could not be compelled to produce . . . if the subsequent proceedings had begun. (By virtue of the County Court Rules 1981 (as amended) (hereafter CCR 1981), Order 13, rule 7(g), this provision also applies to claims likely to be begun in the County Court.)

2 The court is prohibited by section 35(1) of the Supreme Court Act 1981 from making an order under section 33(2) if it considers that 'compliance with the order, if made, would be likely to be injurious to the public interest'. (For County Court equivalent *see* section 54(1), County Courts Act 1984). Each of these exceptions will be considered in turn.

Legal professional privilege

The courts consider that they have an overriding obligation to promote full and candid disclosure by clients to their legal advisers. Such disclosure would be impossible if clients feared that communications with their legal advisers were subject to disclosure. Any direct communications between lawyer and client made for the purposes of giving or receiving legal advice are, therefore, privileged from disclosure, irrespective of whether or not legal proceedings have begun or are even contemplated. The principle applies equally to communications between employers and salaried solicitors employed directly by them (*Customs & Excise Commissioners v. Alfred Crompton Amusement Machines Ltd* [1972] 2 QB 102).

However, reports prepared by a third party, as is often the case with accident reports, will only enjoy privilege from disclosure if litigation was contemplated when they were written. Moreover, where the report was prepared for more than one reason, its submission to the hospital or health authority solicitor in anticipation of litigation must be at least the dominant purpose for which it was prepared.

In the leading case of *Waugh v. British Railways Board* [1980] Ac 521, the plaintiff's husband, an employee of the British Railways Board, was killed in an accident while working on the railways. In accordance with the Board's usual practice, an internal enquiry report was prepared by two of the Board's officers two days after the accident. The report was headed 'For the information of the Board's solicitor', but it was admitted that the report was prepared for two purposes: to establish the cause of the accident so that appropriate safety measures could be taken; and to enable the Board's solicitor to advise in the litigation that was likely to follow. Although the first purpose was more immediate than the second, they were described by the Board as being of equal importance. The plaintiff applied to the court for discovery of the report to assist in the preparation and conduct of her case, but the Board resisted the application on the grounds that the report was protected by legal professional privilege.

The court was faced with two conflicting principles. On the one hand, all relevant evidence should be made available to the court; and on the other, communications between lawyer and client should remain confidential. In reconciling these two principles their lordships held that on balance the public interest was best served by confining within narrow limits the privilege of lawfully withholding relevant evidence.

> Justice is better served by candour than by suppression. For as it was put in *Grant v. Downs* [135 CLR 647 at 686] . . . 'the privilege . . . detracts from the fairness of the trial by denying a party access to relevant documents or at least subjecting him to surprise'. Lord Edmund-Davies at page 543d

A document will, therefore, only be privileged from production if the main purpose for its preparation was that of submitting it to a legal adviser for advice and use in litigation. Since the preparation of the internal enquiry report for advice and use in litigation was merely one of the purposes, and not the dominant purpose for which it was prepared, the Board's claim to privilege failed. Their lordships added that the fact that the report stated on its face that it was (finally) to be sent to the Board's solicitors, was not conclusive in showing it to be the dominant purpose behind its preparation.

The decision was applied to a health authority accident report in *Lask v. Gloucester Health Authority (The Times,* 13 December 1985). The Court of Appeal held that a confidential accident report which NHS circulars required to be completed by health authorities, both for the use of solicitors in the event of litigation and also to enable action to be taken to avoid a repetition of the accident, was not subject to legal professional privilege. Although the health authority and the solicitors had sworn affidavits that the dominant purpose of its commission was for submission to the solicitors in anticipation of litigation and, despite the report itself referring only to that purpose, the court, after examining the wording of the relevant health circular, decided otherwise.

Public interest immunity

The courts will not order the discovery of documents where to do so would be injurious to the public interest. Immunity from disclosure is most frequently to be found in respect of documents concerning the formulation of government policy, the functioning of a public service, or police or similar investigations. However, it may be possible for a claim of public interest immunity to be made where the applicant seeks access to the medical records of a third party.

> 'Confidentiality' is not a separate head of privilege, but it may be a very material consideration to bear in mind when privilege is claimed on the ground of public interest. What the court has to do is to weigh on the one hand the considerations which suggest that it is in the public interest that the documents in question should be disclosed and on the other hand those which suggest that it is in the public interest that they should not be disclosed and to balance one against the other. Lord Cross, *Alfred Crompton Amusement Machines Ltd v. Customs and Excise Commissioners (No. 2)* [1974] AC 405 at page 433H

Whether the public interest favouring the disclosure of medical records will outweigh the public interest in preserving their confidentiality, will depend upon the particular facts of each case. Nevertheless, the leading case of *Campbell v. Tameside Metropolitan Borough Council* [1982] 1 QB 1065 provides a useful illustration of the approach that a court is likely to take.

The applicant, a school teacher employed by the defendant education authority, was violently assaulted by a pupil. Her legal advisers believed that she might have a claim against her employers for negligence in failing to transfer the pupil to a special school for maladjusted children. Before deciding whether or not to bring proceedings, her advisers wished to see whether the reports of other teachers, education psychologists and psychiatrists showed him to be of so violent a disposition that he would be a danger at an ordinary school. The authority contended that the documents were confidential and protected from disclosure by public interest immunity. However, on inspection of the documents, the Court of Appeal held that they were of considerable significance and as such, the public interest favoured disclosure.

> There is no difference between this case and other school cases where a child is injured in the playground by defective equipment, or by want of supervision by the teacher. Full discovery would be ordered there. There is no difference in principle between a child being injured and a teacher being injured. Nor indeed do I see any difference between this case and the ordinary case against a hospital for negligence. The reports of doctors and

nurses are, of course, confidential; but they must always be disclosed: subject to the safeguard that they are only for use in connection with the instant case and not for any other purpose. Lord Denning, Master of the Rolls, at 1074G

A similar approach was taken in *Flett v. North Tameside Health Authority* [1990] CLY 2968. The plaintiff, a nurse who had been injured while lifting an obese and partially disabled patient, successfully obtained an order for the disclosure of the patient's medical records. The court held that the case was analogous to an industrial accident where any records concerning the size, shape and weight of the component would be disclosed. The fact that the documents in the present case were confidential was not in itself sufficient to justify their being withheld.

It appears, therefore, that in relation to medical records, a claim of public interest immunity is only likely to succeed where the documents are of little significance to the contemplated litigation or where there is some additional factor favouring the preservation of confidentiality. An example of the circumstances in which a claim of public interest immunity will be upheld is provided by *D v. National Society for the Prevention of Cruelty to Children* [1978] AC 171. The Society received a complaint from an informant about the treatment of a 14-month-old girl. An inspector was sent to the parents' home to investigate the allegation. The mother subsequently brought an action against the Society, alleging that the Society had acted negligently in their investigation which, she claimed, caused her severe and continuing shock. During the course of the litigation the Society sought to withhold disclosure of any documents which would reveal the identity of the informant. The House of Lords upheld the Society's argument on the basis that if disclosure were ordered then the Society's sources of information would dry up and this would be contrary to the public interest.

Where it is sought to rely on public interest immunity, the party invoking the immunity must establish that the public interest is clearly best served by withholding disclosure:

[T]he question to be determined is whether it is clearly demonstrated that in the particular case the public interest would nevertheless be better served by excluding evidence despite its relevance. If, on balance, the matter is left in doubt, disclosure should be ordered. Lord Edmund-Davies, *D v. NSPCC* (above) at page 246D

Should it be necessary, the court may order that the documents for which immunity from discovery is claimed, should be produced at court so a decision can be made as to whether disclosure would, in fact, be contrary to the public interest.

The grounds for discovery

The following grounds for discovery apply equally to applications for discovery against health service bodies (ie NHS Trusts, district and regional health authorities) as they do to applications against general practitioners. References to 'health service bodies' may, therefore, be taken as including reference to general practitioners unless the contrary is stated.

1 The applicant must be 'likely to be a party to subsequent proceedings'

The applicant will in the vast majority of cases be a patient contemplating bringing proceedings against the health service body. However, all that is required is that he or she be likely to be a party to subsequent proceedings. For example, where a patient has sustained an injury while undergoing treatment in two different districts, he or she will be able to seek discovery of the notes held by each authority in order to determine the likely source of the injury. Each authority may also then seek pre-action discovery of the notes held by the other, so as to enable a defence to be prepared at the earliest possible opportunity.

Does the applicant have to show that at the time of the application he or she has sufficient evidence on which to base a claim, in order to establish that proceedings are 'likely'?

No. This argument was unsuccessful in the leading case *Dunning v. Board of Governors of the United Liverpool Hospitals* [1973] 2 All ER 454.

In 1963, Mrs Dunning, who had enjoyed good health all her life, developed a persistent cough and was admitted to hospital for investigation. After two or three weeks her condition became dramatically worse and when she was finally discharged from hospital, some 17 weeks after her admission, her illness had not cleared up. She was initially diagnosed as suffering from undulant fever but finally from *periarteritis nodosa*. However, her family took the view that her condition had been caused by one of the drugs given to her in hospital. Even so, no action was taken against the hospital within the limitation period, probably because Mrs Dunning's doctor had told her that her condition would clear up. Any action would therefore have become statute-barred unless the court granted leave to sue out of time because of the applicant's ignorance of material facts.

In 1969, Mrs Dunning, who had still not recovered, was granted legal aid to ascertain whether there were grounds for applying for leave to bring an action for negligence against the hospital Board out of time. Mrs Dunning's medical adviser, Dr Evans, then sought access to the hospital case notes. However, the Board was unwilling to make them available unless it received an assurance that no action would be taken against it; an assurance which Mrs Dunning's solicitors declined to give.

In May 1970, without having seen the notes, Dr Evans formed the opinion that, on the evidence available to him, the hospital had not acted negligently. As his opinion disclosed no real basis for a claim, nothing more happened until section 31 of the Administration Act 1970 came into force (the relevant wording of which is identical to that of the present section 33(2)). The Board was ordered by Mr Justice Caulfield to make the records available to Dr Evans, but appealed.

In the Court of Appeal, counsel for the Board argued that the plain wording of the section empowered the Court to order discovery only if the applicant could show that at the time of the application she was likely to bring a claim in respect of her illness, and that the report of Dr Evans had advised that there was no foundation for making any such claim. Disclosure was therefore being sought, counsel argued, not for the purpose of providing evidence on which a claim could be based, but merely to allay the anxieties of Mrs Dunning and her family. Accordingly, he submitted, discovery should be refused.

The court rejected the submission (Lord Justice Stamp dissenting). Lord Denning, Master of the Rolls, and Lord Justice James stated that one of the objects of the section was to enable potential plaintiffs to find out whether there is evidence upon which to bring a claim before incurring the expense of commencing proceedings. The purpose of the legislation would be frustrated if the applicant had to show in advance of seeing her medical records, that she had already had sufficient evidence upon which to base her claim.

> I think that we should construe 'likely to be made' as meaning 'may' or 'may well be made' dependent on the outcome of discovery. Lord Denning, Master of the Rolls, at page 475f

The question for the court is, therefore, whether the applicant is likely to commence proceedings if the notes disclose evidence of negligence, which in Mrs Dunning's case was 'reasonably certain'. Accordingly, an order for discovery was granted.

However, pre-action discovery does not permit an aggrieved patient simply to go on a 'fishing expedition' for evidence of negligence. He or she must disclose the nature of the proposed claim, and show not only that he or she intends to make it, but also that there is a reasonable basis for doing so:

> Illfounded, irresponsible and speculative allegations based merely on hope would not provide a reasonable basis for an intended claim in subsequent proceedings. Lord Justice James at page 460e

The applicant has to establish that he or she is 'likely' to bring proceedings against the health service body if the notes disclose evidence of negligence. Does this mean 'more probable than not?'

No. In *Harris v. Newcastle upon Tyne Health Authority* [1989] 1 WLR 96, Sir John Megaw accepted that the ordinary and sensible meaning of the word 'likely' involves something which is not unlikely, which in turn is something which is more probable than not. However, his Lordship added:

> On the authority of this Court in *Dunning v. United Liverpool Hospital Board of Governors* . . ..I have come to the conculsion that we are bound by that authority to construe the word 'likely' . . . as having the meaning which James LJ gave to it when he said: 'I would construe "likely" . . . as meaning "reasonable prospect".' You can have a reasonable prospect even though you may fall considerably short of more than a 50% chance. Another phrase which might be used to describe the same effect is . . . 'on the cards'. (at 279C)

2 The claim must be 'in respect of personal injury or death'

'Personal injury' is defined by section 35 of the Act as including 'any disease and any impairment of a person's physical or mental condition'.

It is important to note that the power to order discovery is not limited to cases where an allegation of medical negligence is likely to be made. Health service bodies may, therefore, find pre-action discovery being sought by, for example, employees injured while at work. Moreover, not every medical negligence claim will necessarily be 'in respect of personal injuries'. For example, the negligent diagnosis of dysfunction in a healthy patient is likely only to cause the patient financial loss by his being advised to give up work for a period of time.[1]

3 The person against whom disclosure is sought must be 'likely to be a party to the proceedings'

Unless the health service body is 'likely to be a party to the proceedings', a patient is not entitled to invoke the section to obtain access to his or her medical notes. This represents an important limitation on the scope of the section; the vast majority of personal injury claims being brought against motorists and employers who have no connection whatsoever with the NHS. However, there is no reason why patients should not be permitted access to their notes in such circumstances, providing that criteria (1) and (2) on page 47 are satisfied.

[1]Lewis CJ, *Medical negligence – a plaintiff's guide*, (page 57), 1988, Frank Cass.

Disclosure must be necessary either to dispose of the case fairly or to save costs

This additional criterion is required by Order 24, rule 8 of the Rules of the Supreme Court, which provides that:

> On the hearing of an application for an order . . . the Court, if satisfied that discovery is not necessary, or not necessary at that stage of the cause or matter, may dismiss or, as the case may be, adjourn the application and shall in any case refuse to make such an order if and so far as it is of the opinion that discovery is not necessary either for disposing fairly of the cause or matter or for saving costs. (By virtue of CCR 1981, Order 13, rule 7(g), this provision also applies to applications made in the County Court.)

It is unlikely that a court will refuse an application for pre-action discovery on the grounds that it is unnecessary, particularly where an allegation of medical negligence may be made.

- As has already been noted, the nature of clinical medicine is such that it will frequently be difficult, if not impossible, to assess whether there is any basis for bringing a claim, without first obtaining access to the patient's notes.
- The courts appear to be increasingly of the opinion that a patient should have a right to be told exactly what treatment he or she has received.

It should not be forgotten that we are concerned here with a hospital-patient relationship. The recent decision of the House of Lords in *Sidaway v. Bethlem Royal Hospital Governors* [1985] 2 WLR 480 affirms that a doctor is under a duty to answer his patient's questions as to the treatment proposed. We see no reason why this should not be a similar duty in relation to hospital staff . . . Why, we ask ourselves, is the position any different if the patient asks what treatment he has in fact had? Let us suppose that a blood transfusion is in contemplation. The patient asks what is involved. He is told that a quantity of blood from a donor will be introduced into his system. He may ask about the risk of AIDS and so forth and will be entitled to straight answers. He consents. Suppose that, by accident, he is given a quantity of air as well as blood and suffers serious ill effects. Is he not entitled to ask what treatment he in fact received, and is the doctor and hospital authority not obliged to tell him, 'In the event you did not only get a blood transfusion. You also got an air transfusion'? Why is the duty different before the treatment from what it is afterwards? Sir John Donaldson, Master of the Rolls, *Lee v. South West Thames Regional Area Health Authority* [1985] 2 All ER 385 at 201J

- Thirdly, the courts are especially reluctant to refuse an order for pre-action discovery where the applicant is legally aided, as will be the case in a significant proportion of applications.

There is an important aspect of the matter which I think it is right for the Court before whom such an application comes to bear in mind. That is the public interest where the plaintiff is qualified for legal aid. Where the plaintiff is qualified for legal aid, his advisers are under a duty to inform the legal aid committee of their view of his prospects of succeeding in the action and to keep the committee informed from time to time throughout the progress of the proceedings of any change in that respect; it is undesirable that proceedings should be brought or continued with legal aid beyond the point at which it is reasonably clear that the plaintiff has no substantial prospect of success; and therefore there is a special ground for saying that the advisers of legally aided parties should have as early information as possible on matters which may affect that aspect of a legally aided party's position in the litigation. Lord Justice Buckley, *Shaw v. Vauxhall Motors* [1974] 1 WLR 1035 at 1040H

Requests for disclosure

Before making a formal application to the court, it is usual and proper first to request that the patient's notes be disclosed voluntarily.

To whom should the request be made?

Where the medication notes sought relate to treatment undertaken in a hospital, the request should be made to the chief executive of the health service body which manages the hospital. This will normally be the local district health authority but may occasionally be the regional health authority. In the case of NHS Trust hospitals, however, the hospital will be self-managed and so the request should be addressed to the chief executive of the hospital. Where the medical records to which access is sought are held by a general practitioner, the request may be made to any member of the practice partnership. As previously noted, references to 'health service bodies' may be taken as also including reference to general practitioners, unless the contrary is stated.

Besides requiring sufficient details to enable the relevant notes to be located, the health service body will not be in a position to process the request unless:

- it states whether proceedings are contemplated against the body, and if so, the grounds on which negligence is alleged or suspected

- a letter of consent signed by the patient authorizing disclosure is included with the request
- the applicant undertakes not to use the records for any other purpose; and
- the applicant undertakes to pay the costs reasonably incurred in dealing with the request.

The health service body's response

An unreasonable refusal may result in the health service body being ordered to pay the costs incurred by the applicant should an application be made to court (*see* Costs, page 50). It will usually be in the health service body's interests to respond to a proper request for discovery by agreeing to disclose the patient's notes voluntarily, provided that:

1 Where the information sought is of a medical nature (occasionally the information sought may be entirely unrelated to medical matters, for example, the date of the patient's admission to, or discharge from, hospital), the doctor or dentist in charge of the patient's treatment, or his or her successor, is consulted in accordance with HM(59)88 (*see* Annex A to HC(82)16, reproduced on pages 168–9). This is to ensure that the notes do not contain information which might harm the patient and that any extracts requested are not misleading. The disclosure of information harmful to the patient, may result in a separate claim being brought against the health service body. Where the patient is legally represented, this problem will usually be overcome by getting an undertaking from his or her solicitor that he or she will not communicate the contents of the notes to the patient. Providing that the reason for seeking to restrict access is explained, such an undertaking will usually be forthcoming.

2 Disclosure will not reveal information concerning, or provided by, an identifiable third party, unless the third party either has consented to the disclosure (preferably in writing), or is a health professional who has provided the information in a professional capacity. Failure to obtain the requisite consent may result in a claim for breach of confidence (*see* Chapter 7), and if the patient's notes are stored on computer, action being taken by the Data Protection Registrar.

Unless the above criteria are satisfied, the patient's notes should not be disclosed voluntarily. Although the applicant may be able to obtain a court order compelling disclosure, where disclosure is ordered by the court the health authority will enjoy immunity from proceedings in respect of the disclosure (*see* Chapter 7, page 76).

Where a patient's notes are to be disclosed, the relevant notes should be copied and the copies placed in an indexed bundle or file (*M v. Plymouth Health Authority, The Times*, 26 November 1992).

To whom should disclosure be made?

In the past, medical defence societies and health authorities alike have sought to limit disclosure to a nominated expert only. While plaintiffs' solicitors are content to accept disclosure to a nominated expert only, the practice will no doubt continue.

Disclosure to a nominated expert only puts plaintiffs' solicitors at a distinct disadvantage. They will not be able to ensure that notes their expert receives are complete and neither they, nor their clients, will be able to direct the expert to any aspect of the notes they regard as significant. If the report is unfavourable, it will be difficult, if not impossible, to detect whether the expert has been less than forthcoming in suggesting areas of potential negligence. Also, should a second opinion be required, the solicitor will be forced to request further disclosure of the patient's notes, thus alerting the defence to the fact that the prosecution has had little success with its first effort. This will hardly encourage the defence to favour an early settlement of the claim.

There is no legal basis for seeking to limit disclosure to a nominated medical adviser only. The Act expressly states that the court may order disclosure:

... to the applicant or, on such conditions as may be specified in the order:

(i)   to the applicant's legal advisers; or
(ii) to the applicant's legal advisers and any other medical or professional adviser of the applicant; or
(iii) if the applicant has no legal adviser, to any medical adviser or other professional adviser of the applicant.

While an order for pre-action discovery may exclude the applicant from being permitted access to his or her notes, so long as a lawyer has been retained the lawyer must be permitted to examine them.

As a result of increasing specialization and experience of medical negligence litigation, few solicitors are now prepared to accept disclosure to a nominated expert only, and will say so when requesting disclosure.

May a charge be made for disclosing a patient's notes voluntarily?

Health authorities are now permitted to fix their own charges for the supply of information about patients involved in legal proceedings (*see* HC(87)13). Any charges made should be limited to recovery of the costs incurred by the authority and should not include an element of profit. There is no reason why NHS Trusts and general practitioners should not similarly charge for the costs they incur.

Applications to court

It is rare for a patient to have to resort to making an application to court in order to obtain discovery of his or her medical records. However, a small number of applications are made each year, and it is worth outlining the procedures involved in making and responding to an application to the court.

An application for an order for pre-action discovery must be made by serving upon the chief executive of the responsible Trust, district or regional health authority, or in the case of a general practitioner, the members of the practice partnership, or any other person authorized to accept service, such as solicitors, an 'originating summons' issued in the High Court (RSC 1965, Order 24, rule 7A(1)). Where it is appropriate to make the application to the County Court (*see* page 37), the application is referred to as an 'originating application'. The procedure for bringing such an application is the same as that for issuing an originating summons in the High Court (CCR 1981, Order 13, rule 7(1)(g)). References to 'originating summons' may, therefore, be taken as also applying to 'originating applications'.

The summons must be supported by an affidavit which must:

(a) . . . state the grounds on which it is alleged that the applicant and the person against whom the order is sought are likely to be parties to subsequent proceedings . . . in which a claim for personal injuries is likely to be made; and

(b) . . . specify or describe the documents in respect of which an order is sought and show . . . that the documents are relevant to an issue arising or likely to arise out of a claim for personal injuries made or likely to be made in the proceedings and that the person against whom the order is sought is likely to have or have had them in his possession, custody or power. (RSC 1965, Order 24, r7A(3))

The health service body's response

The summons must be acknowledged by properly completing the 'acknowledgement of service' which accompanies the summons. The acknowledgement of service must be returned to the court within 14 days (RSC 1965, Order 12, rule 9). The date of service is included in the 14 days.

Costs

Even where an application for pre-action discovery is successful, it is by no means certain that proceedings against the defendant will follow, the applicant merely having to establish that there is a 'reasonable prospect' of subsequent proceedings. It is therefore inappropriate for an order for costs to be 'reserved' to the trial judge. Irrespective of whether or not the application is successful, the defendant will usually be entitled to an order that the applicant pays the costs that he or she has incurred.

Where the applicant is legally aided, an order that the applicant pay the defendant's costs will not be enforceable without leave of the court, which will rarely be forthcoming. Furthermore, the court's power to order the legal aid board to pay costs is seriously curtailed. Under the Legal Aid Act 1988, a court may only grant such an order where:

- an order for cost would have been made anyway (ie had the plaintiff not been legally aided)
- the proceedings were instituted by the legally-aided party
- the unassisted party would suffer 'severe financial hardship' unless the order is made; and
- it is just and equitable to make an award for costs out of public funds.

The need to establish 'severe financial hardship', in practice, bars defence societies and health service bodies alike from recovering their costs (*see Hanning v. Maitland (No. 2)* [1970] 1 QB 580).

The court may refuse to grant an order for costs where the health service body in question has been dilatory in complying with a proper request for discovery. A period of six weeks within which to consent to disclosure, and a further 14 days within which to produce the notes, was approved of in *Hall and Others v. Wandsworth Health Authority* [1985] 129 SJ 188. If, for a particular reason, this is insufficient, the defendant should request more time, preferably with an explanation, in order to avoid being refused an award of costs.

Where there is no reasonable basis for refusing discovery, the court may even order that the health service body pay the applicant's costs (*see Hall and Others v. Wandsworth Health Authority* (above), and *Jacob (A Minor) v. Wessex Regional Health Authority* [1984] CLY 2618).

Enforcement

Any person failing to comply with an order for discovery is liable to committal for contempt of court (RSC 1965 0.24, r16(2)).

5

Access During Legal Proceedings

Introduction

As we have already seen, patients bringing personal injury claims may require access to their medical records. However, relevant parts of these records may be exempt from the access provisions of the Data Protection Act 1984, and the Access to Health Records Act 1990. Furthermore, unless a patient is contemplating bringing a claim against the health service body that holds the relevant records, the courts are not empowered to order disclosure before proceedings have been commenced (*see* Chapter 4, page 45). However, once he has actually commenced proceedings by issuing a writ, the court may order disclosure. The power to do so is contained in section 34(2) of the Supreme Court Act 1981 which provides:

> On the application, in accordance with the rules of court, of a party to any proceedings to which this section applies, the High Court shall, in such circumstances as may be specified in the rules, have power to order a person who is not a party to the proceedings and who appears to the court to be likely to have in his possession, custody or power any documents which are relevant to an issue arising out of the said claim:
>
> (a) to disclose whether those documents are in his possession, custody or power; and
> (b) to produce such of those documents, as are in his possession, custody or power to the applicant or, on such conditions as may be specified in the order.

In respect of claims where damages are likely to be less than £50 000 and so are brought in the County Court, the County Court has the same powers as the High Court to order the disclosure of documents (Section 53, County Courts Act 1984). Any references to the powers of the High Court may therefore be taken as also including the powers of the County Court.

Which records are covered by the section?

As with 'pre-action' discovery, the section empowers the court to disclose any relevant documents other than those protected by legal professional privilege (RSC 1965 Order 24, rule 7A(6)), or public interest immunity (section 35(1), Supreme Court Act 1981) (*see* pages 38–41).

The grounds for discovery

1 *The applicant must be a party to present legal proceedings*
It is important to note that the applicant need not be the plaintiff. The section, therefore, permits a defendant to obtain access to the plaintiff's records where, for example, he or she disputes the extent of the plaintiff's alleged injuries.

2 *The health service body must not be a party to the proceedings*
The section empowers the court to order the disclosure of documents only against a person who is not a party to the litigation. Where a person has commenced proceedings against a health service body, he or she will be precluded from obtaining access to his or her medical records under the section.

It will be rare for a person who has commenced proceedings against a health service body to require access to the medical records, it being usual to obtain disclosure of the records before commencing proceedings. If, however, there has been a significant delay between the time when the allegedly negligent treatment was administered and the time when the patient is seeking legal advice, a writ may have to be issued immediately so that the action does not become time-barred. Occasionally, health service bodies may therefore receive requests for disclosure on behalf of a patient who has already commenced proceedings against it. In such circumstances, the court may order the disclosure of the records under Order 24, rule 7 of the Rules of the Supreme Court which states that:

> The Court may at any time, on the application of any party to a cause or matter, make an order requiring any other party to make an affidavit stating whether he has any document specified or described in the application or any class of document so specified or described that is, or at any time has been, in his possession, custody or power.

Although the rule does not specifically refer to the disclosure of documents, it is accepted in practice that the court does have jurisdiction to enforce an order where appropriate. Where it has not been possible to make an application for pre-action discovery, the court will usually be sympathetic to an application under RSC 1965, Order 24, rule 7, provided that there is a reasonable basis for bringing the claim.

3 The claim must be in respect of personal injuries or death

The scope of section 34(2) is significantly curtailed by subsection 1 which states that the power to order disclosure applies only to claims:

> . . . made in respect of personal injuries to a person, or in respect of a person's death.

However, the words 'in respect of' are significant. For the purposes of the section, it is sufficient if the personal injuries have some connection with the plaintiff's claim, even if the claim itself is not for those injuries. For example, in *Patterson v. Chadwick* [1974] 1 WLR 890, the plaintiff had instructed solicitors to act on her behalf in connection with a claim for medical negligence. When the solicitors failed to commence proceedings against the hospital before her claim became time-barred, the plaintiff then began proceedings against her former solicitors for negligence and breach of contract, and sought disclosure of her hospital records to assist her in the claim. Mr Justice Boreham held that the words 'in respect of' conveyed the need for some connection or relation between the plaintiff's claim and the personal injuries that she had sustained, and that since the nature and extent of her personal injuries formed an essential ingredient in the proof of her claim agianst her former solicitors, that connection was present.

4 Disclosure must be necessary either to dispose of the case fairly, or to save costs

This additional criterion is required by Order 24, rule 8 of the Rules of the Supreme Court (*see* page 45). In the majority of cases it is necessary to obtain the patient's medication notes, to determine either liability or more usually quantum (damages). It is therefore unusual for a court to refuse an application for disclosure on the basis that it is unnecessary, either to dispose of the case fairly or to save costs, particularly where the applicant is legally aided (*see* page 46).

Requests for disclosure

Before making a formal application to the court, it is usual and proper first to request that the patient's notes be disclosed voluntarily. In the case of hospital notes, the person to whom to address the request is not the responsible consultant but the chief executive of the responsible health service body. (For a discussion of the responsible health service body, *see* page 46.) In the case of notes held by a general practitioner, the request should be addressed to that practitioner or any other member of the partnership. (Hereafter, references to 'health service bodies' may be taken as also including reference to general practitioners unless the contrary is stated.)

Besides requiring sufficient details to enable the relevant notes to be located, the appropriate health service body will not be in a position to process the request unless:

- it briefly outlines the nature of the claim
- a letter of consent signed by the patient authorizing disclosure is included with the request
- an undertaking is given not to use the records for any other purpose; and
- the applicant undertakes to pay the costs reasonably incurred in dealing with the request.

The health service body's response

An unreasonable refusal to disclose a patient's notes may ultimately result in the health service body being ordered to pay the costs incurred by the applicant should an application be made to the court (*see* page 47). It will usually be in the health service body's interests to respond to a proper request for disclosure by agreeing to disclose the notes voluntarily, provided that:

1 Where the information sought is of a medical nature (occasionally the information sought may be entirely unrelated to medical matters, for example, the date of the patient's admission to, or discharge from hospital), the doctor or dentist in charge of the patient's treatment, or his or her successor, is consulted in accordance with HM(59)88 (*see* Annex A to HC(82)16, pages 168–9). This is to ensure that the notes do not contain information which might harm the patient and that any extracts requested are not misleading. The disclosure of information harmful to the patient may result in a claim being brought against the health authority. Where the patient is legally represented, this problem will usually be overcome by getting an undertaking from his or her representative that he or she will not communicate the contents of the notes to the patient. Providing that the reason for seeking to restrict access is explained, such an undertaking will usually be forthcoming.

2 Disclosure will not reveal information concerning or provided by an identifiable third party, unless the third party either has consented to the disclosure (preferably in writing) or is a health professional who has provided the information in a professional capacity. Failure to obtain

the requisite consent may result in a claim for breach of confidence (*see* Chapter 7), and if the patient's notes are stored on computer, action being taken by the Data Protection Registrar.

Unless both criteria are satisfied, the patient's notes should not be disclosed. Although the applicant may be able to obtain a court order compelling disclosure, where disclosure is ordered by a court, the health service body will enjoy immunity from proceedings in respect of the disclosure (*see* Chapter 7, page 76).

To whom should disclosure be made?

The Act states that the court may order disclosure:

> . . . to the applicant or, on such conditions as may be specified in the order:
> (i)   to the applicant's legal advisers; or
> (ii) to the applicant's legal advisers and any other medical or professional adviser of the applicant; or
> (iii) if the applicant has no legal adviser, to any medical adviser or other professional adviser of the applicant.

Whilst an order for discovery may exclude the applicant from being permitted access to his or her notes, as long as a legal adviser has been retained, the adviser must be permitted to examine the notes. There is no legal basis for seeking to limit disclosure to a nominated medical expert only.

May a charge be made for disclosing a patient's notes voluntarily?

Health authorities are now permitted to fix their own charges for the supply of information about patients involved in legal proceedings (*see* HC(87)13). Any charges made should be limited to recovery of the costs incurred by the authority and should not include an element of profit. There is no reason why NHS Trusts and general practitioners should not also make such a charge.

Applications to court

An application for discovery must be made by serving a summons on the chief executive (or any person authorized to accept service, such as authority solicitors) and on every party to the proceedings (Order 24, rule 7A(2)). Where the proceedings have been brought in the County Court, the application is referred to as an application 'by notice' (CCR 1981, Order 13, rule 7(4)). The procedure for bringing such an application is the same as that for issuing a summons in the High Court (CCR 1981, Order 13, rule 7(1)(g)). References to 'summons' may, therefore, be taken as also applying to 'notice'.

The summons must be supported by an affidavit which must:

> . . . specify or describe the documents in respect of which the order is sought and show . . . that the documents are relevant to an issue arising or likely to arise out of a claim for personal injuries . . . and that the person against whom the order is sought is likely to have or have had them in his possession, custody or power. (RSC 1965, Order 24, rule 7A(3)(b))

Again, a copy of the affidavit must be served on every party to the proceedings.

The health service body's response

The summons must be acknowledged by properly completing the 'acknowledgement of service' which accompanies the summons. The acknowledgement of service must be returned to the court within 14 days (RSC 1965, Order 12, rule 9). The date of service is included in the 14 days.

Costs

Since the health service body is not a party to the claim, but has temporarily been brought into the proceedings by a party seeking access to (usually) their medical records, the body will normally be entitled to an order that the applicant pay its costs. Where the applicant is legally aided, it is highly unlikely that the order will be enforceable. Furthermore, the court may deny the body its costs if in some way it has been at fault or even, in exceptional cases, order that it pay the applicant's costs. (For a full discussion of costs *see* Chapter 4, page 50.)

Enforcement

Any person failing to comply with an order for discovery is liable to commital for contempt of court (RSC 1965 Order 24, rule 16(2)).

6

Access to Medical Reports

Introduction

In any personal injury claim it will be necessary to obtain a medical report concerning the plaintiff's present and future prognosis, a copy of which must be served on the defendant along with the summons or writ commencing the action (RSC 1965, Order 18, rule 12(1A), CCR 1981, Order 6, rule 1(5)). If medical evidence is relevant to liability, for example in medical negligence claims, or the extent of the plaintiff's injuries is in dispute, further medical evidence will need to be obtained by both sides for use in the trial. The plaintiff will therefore have to undergo further examinations by both sides' medical experts (a refusal to be examined by the defendant's expert would normally result in his or her claim being 'stayed', thereby preventing it from being further prosecuted). Where such expert reports are commissioned, each party will wish to obtain access to the other's report. This prevents either party from conducting their case in ignorance of the strength of the other's, which in turn promotes an early settlement or, should the case proceed to trial, enables the issues in the case to be defined in advance, saving time and expense. To this end, the Rules of Court provide for the disclosure of such reports. However, the Rules differ depending upon whether the claim is brought in the County Court or High Court and, if brought in the High Court, whether the claim involves an allegation of medical negligence.

Claims brought in the High Court

Personal injury claims (not involving medical negligence)

Before a matter goes to trial, the issues involved have to be identified by the parties in the form of documents, referred to as 'pleadings', which set out the nature of the claim and the defence. In personal injury claims, other than those involving an allegation of medical negligence, automatic directions take effect 14 days after the pleadings are deemed to be closed (pleadings are deemed to be closed 14 days after a defence has been served on the plaintiff). These directions require, *inter alia*, that:

> where any party intends to place reliance at the trial . . . on expert evidence, he shall, within 14 weeks, disclose the substance of that evidence to the other parties in the form of a written report. (RSC 1965, Order 15, rule 8(b))

The rules further provide that the reports shall be disclosed by mutual exchange, each party sending the substance of its expert evidence to the other at the same time (RSC Order 25, rule 8(2)). In this way neither party gains a tactical advantage from seeing the other's evidence before they finalize their own.

It is important to note that the directions only require that each party disclose the substance of the evidence which they intend to rely on at trial. Neither party is obliged to disclose the contents of a report which proves to be unfavourable to their case, provided that they do not intend to call the author as an expert witness or intend to rely on the report at trial.

Does the court have the power to order that different directions should apply?

Yes. Paragraph 3 of the Order (above) entitles either party to apply to court 'for such further or different directions or orders as may, in the circumstances, be appropriate'. For example, if it is highly impractical or unduly expensive for one party to instruct their own expert to prepare a report, until it is known what precise contentions will be put forward by the opposing party, it may be appropriate to apply for 'sequential' disclosure.

Any application under paragraph 3 must be justified on proper grounds. Failure to justify the application, for example, where the applicant simply intends to delay the progress of the claim, will almost certainly result in an order to pay the costs incurred by the other party in opposing the application.

Can the plaintiff demand that, as a condition of submitting to an examination by the defendant's doctor, he be entitled to see the report?

Should the defendant's solicitor agree to such a condition, then the court will, if necessary, order that the report be disclosed. However, the defendant's solicitor will rarely make such a concession and, should the plaintiff continue to insist that the ensuing report must be disclosed, he or she will almost certainly apply to have the plaintiff's action 'stayed', so preventing the claim from being further prosecuted. The court will only 'stay' the plaintiff's claim if it is established that the plaintiff's refusal to submit to the examination is unreasonable. The onus of establishing unreasonableness is on the defendant. However, the courts have clearly stated that, save perhaps in exceptional circumstances, the plaintiff is not entitled to impose such a condition upon the defendant.

> It is perfectly easy to understand the plaintiff's feelings and his wish to know what the defendants' doctor has said about him; and in terms of ordinary human response that is perfectly comprehensible and quite natural. But the question here is whether in litigation it is fair and just not only to the plaintiff but to both sides. It means quite clearly that the plaintiff, if he is right, can insist on seeing a copy of the defendants' doctor's medical report as a condition of submitting to the medical examination, and if that report is more favourable to his case than his own doctor's, he can call, or be in a position to call, that doctor if so advised. That might be sound enough in terms of fairness, but the corollary is that he, the plaintiff, should disclose all medical reports which he has obtained even if they are unfavourable to his case. I should image that most plaintiffs and their advisers would think that that was a major encroachment on the privileges of a litigant in these courts. Lord Justice Ormrod, *Megarity v. D J Ryan & Sons Ltd* [1980] 2 All ER 832 at 836f

Sanctions for non-compliance

Failure to comply with the automatic directions of Order 25 rule 8 can have serious consequences. The defaulting party loses the right to call the expert as a witness at trial or to put the expert's report in evidence, having to obtain either the other party's consent or the leave of the court to do so (RSC 1965, Order 38, rule 36(1)). Whether the court will grant leave to cite expert evidence will depend upon the facts of the case. However, leave will probably not be given if the party has deliberately refrained from complying with the rules so as to gain a tactical advantage. If non-compliance with the rules was unintended, leave will probably be granted if the court thinks it necessary to dispose fairly of the case, but the defaulting party can expect to be ordered to pay any costs incurred by the default (it may be necessary, for example, to adjourn the case in order to enable the opposing party to consider a reply to the evidence).

Medical negligence claims

Automatic directions do not take effect in the High Court where the claim involves 'an allegation of a negligent act or omission in the course of medical treatment' (RSC 1965, Order 25, rule 8(5)(b)). Instead, any party to the claim must, if he or she intends to call expert evidence at the trial, apply to the court to determine whether the substance of the evidence should be disclosed under RSC 1965, Order 38, rule 7 (RSC 1965, Order 36, rule 36(1)(a), as amended by RSC (Amendment No. 4) 1989 (SI 1989 No. 2427)). This provides that:

> . . . unless the court considers that there are special reasons for not doing so, it shall direct that the substance of the evidence be disclosed in the form of a written report or reports to such other parties and within such period as the court may specify.

It remains to be seen exactly what circumstances will be taken by a court to constitute special reasons for not ordering disclosure. However, in light of observations by the Court of Appeal in *Naylor v. Preston Area Health Authority and other appeals* [1987] 2 All ER 353, it is clear that the court will be slow to find such reasons:

> Justice is not achieved by a war of attrition in which survival is a prize to be awarded to the party with the greatest determination and longest purse. Nor is justice achieved by a surprise attack . . . [N]owadays, the general rule is that, whilst a party is entitled to privacy in seeking out the 'cards' for his hand, once he has put his hand together, most of the cards have to be put down well before the hearing. This is not the product of a change of fashion or even a recognition that professional judges approach their duties on the basis of mental equipment, training and attitudes of mind which are far removed from those of juries. It is the product of a growing appreciation that the public interest demands that justice be provided as swiftly and as economically as possible. Sir John Donaldson, Master of the Rolls, at 359–360

Circumstances in which the court might be prepared to refuse to order disclosure were discussed by Sir Frederick Lawton, although he pointed out that it was not easy to envisage such circumstances applying:

> By way of example only, I suggest the following: disclosure might enable the plaintiff, or his medical experts, to trim their evidence; but this is only likely to happen if there is a substantial dispute about primary facts or there is a reason to think that the plaintiff's medical experts have mistakenly based their opinion on clinical findings which the defendants can prove, or think they can prove, were wrong. Another type of case is that in which the defendants are in possession of evidence, referred to in the expert medical reports, which goes to show that the plaintiff is alleging that he is suffering from a non-existent disability or is exaggerating his symptoms or that his disability is due to an earlier trauma which he has not disclosed. The value of such evidence would be lost if the plaintiff became aware of it before trial. *Naylor v. Preston AHA* at 367

As is the case with automatic directions in other personal injury actions, the Court of Appeal in *Naylor v. Preston AHA* took the view that disclosure should normally be mutual, although it might be prepared to order sequential disclosure in special cases (*see* page 58).

It is important to note that each party may only be required to disclose the substance of the evidence which they intend to rely on at trial. Neither party is obliged to disclose the contents of a report which proves to be unfavourable to their case, provided they do not intend to call the author as an expert witness or intend to rely on the report at trial.

Sanctions for non-compliance
Failure to apply for directions or to comply with those directions has the same consequences as failing to comply with automatic directions under Order 25, rule 8 (*see* page 59).

Claims brought in the County Court

Where any award of damages is likely to be less than £50 000, the claim will be brought in the County Court. The County Court Rules do not distinguish between claims which involve an allegation of medical negligence, and those which do not. Automatic directions requiring the disclosure of expert medical reports will take effect in all personal injury claims in the same way that automatic directions take effect in the High Court, except that the substance of the evidence must be disclosed within 10 and not 14 weeks from the close of pleadings (CCR 1981, Order 17, rule 11). (*See* page 57: Claims brought in the High Court: personal injury claims (not involving medical negligence).)

Access to expert medical reports and the Access to Health Records Act 1990

To obtain access to all the medical reports commissioned by the defendants, and not just the substance of those reports which they intended to rely upon at trial, would be a significant tactical advantage for the plaintiff and his or her advisers. Not only might it alert the plaintiff to any weaknesses in the defendant's case, but should any of the reports be more favourable than those of his or her own experts, the plaintiff could call the author as a witness at trial. It could be argued that the Access to Health Records Act 1990 enables the plaintiff (or the plaintiff's adviser) to do just that by applying directly to the expert for a copy of the report, provided that the report was prepared after 1 November 1991. Unlike the Data Protection Act 1984, which applies to computerized medical records, a claim of legal professional privilege may not entitle the holder of the report to withhold disclosure (*see* Chapter 2).

Professional Confidence and Third Party Access

7

Professional Confidence and Disclosure

The duty of confidence

The duty of confidence owed by a doctor to his or her patients is probably as old as the practice of medicine itself, and is widely regarded as one of the cornerstones of the doctor-patient relationship. This ethical duty has been recognized at least since the time of Hippocrates and is expressly mentioned in his celebrated Oath:

> Whatever, in connection with my professional practice, or not in connection with it, I see or hear in the life of men, which ought not to be spoken abroad, I will not divulge, as reckoning that all such should be kept secret.

It is equally well-established that a doctor owes his or her patient a legal, as well as ethical, obligation of confidence. It is not, however, an absolute duty; there are exceptional cases in which a doctor is legally entitled and, in certain instances, legally obliged to disclose confidential information. The problem lies in identifying these exceptions and determining their scope. Useful guidance is to be found in the General Medical Council's (GMC's) 'Blue Book'.[1] The following list of exceptions draws upon the GMC's advice.

The exceptions

1 Disclosure with the patient's consent

The doctor may be released from his or her obligation of confidence by the express or implied consent of the patient. This is reflected by the first exception to be found in the revised GMC guidance:

> Where a patient, or a person authorised to act on a patient's behalf, consents to the disclosure, information to which the consent refers may be disclosed in accordance with that consent. (para 2)

---

[1]*Professional conduct and discipline: fitness to practise*, 1991, General Medical Council.

In law, the consent need not be in writing in order to be valid. However, given the often sensitive nature of the contents of medical records, it is advisable to require written authorization from the patient whenever possible.

2 Disclosure to other registered medical practitioners and healthcare professionals involved in the care of the individual

The legal justification, for sharing confidential information with other healthcare professionals, is that the patient may be presumed to give his or her consent to such disclosures. This forms the basis of the second exception to be found in the GMC's revised guidance:

> Most doctors in hospital and general practice are working in health care teams, some of whose members may need access to information, given or obtained in confidence about individuals, in order to perform their duties . . . The doctor also has a responsibility to ensure that arrangements exist to inform patients of the circumstances in which information about them is likely to be shared and the opportunity to state any objection to this. (para 4)

Where confidential information is shared with others, and they know or ought to know of the confidential nature of the information, they will be equally bound by the obligation of confidence (*Prince Albert v. Strange* [1849] 1 Mac & G 25).

The patient may expressly state that he or she does not wish particular confidential information to be shared with anyone else at all. Unless the patient can be persuaded otherwise, disclosure to other members of staff cannot be justified on the basis of implied consent. In such circumstances, any disclosure to other healthcare professionals must be justified on other grounds.

3 Disclosure in the patient's best interests

In the course of medical treatment, it may be in the best interests of the patient to disclose confidential information without his or her consent. This is recognized by the seventh, eighth and ninth paragraphs of the GMC's revised guidance.

> In exceptional circumstances a doctor may consider it undesirable, for medical reasons, to seek a patient's consent to the disclosure of confidential information. In such circumstances information may be disclosed

to a relative or some other person, but only when the doctor is satisfied that it is necessary in the patient's medical interests to do so.

Deciding whether or not to disclose information is particularly difficult in cases where a patient cannot be judged capable of giving or withholding consent to disclosure. One such situation may arise where a doctor believes that a patient may be the victim of physical or sexual abuse. In such circumstances the patient's medical interests are paramount and may require the doctor to disclose information to an appropriate person or authority.

Difficulties may also arise when a patient, by reason of immaturity, does not have sufficient understanding to appreciate what the treatment or advice being sought may involve. Similar problems may arise where a patient lacks understanding because of illness or mental incapacity. In all such cases the doctor should attempt to persuade the patient to allow an appropriate person to be involved in the consultation. If the patient cannot understand or be persuaded, but the doctor is convinced that the disclosure of information would be essential to the patient's best medical interests, the doctor may disclose to an appropriate person or authority the fact of the consultation and the information learned in it. A doctor who decides to disclose information must be prepared to justify that decision and must inform the patient before any disclosure is made.

The courts will almost certainly accept that, in certain circumstances, disclosure of confidential information may be justified on the grounds that the disclosure is in the patient's best interests. However, the scope of the exception is particularly unclear, there being no English authority on the point. The approach of the courts is likely to depend upon whether the patient is an adult or child and whether he or she is competent or unable to consent to treatment.

The competent adult

Any doctor who discloses confidential information with the sole justification that it is in the patient's best interests to do so, faces the possibility of an action for breach of confidence. The courts have in the past expressly stated that treatment cannot be imposed on a competent adult patient without his or her consent, irrespective of whether or not the treatment is in the patient's best interests. By analogy, it is unlikely that the courts will permit confidential information concerning a patient to be disclosed solely on the grounds that the doctor considers the disclosure to be in the patient's best interests.

The incompetent adult

Where an adult patient is incapable of consenting to treatment, the doctor responsible for the patient is under a duty to act in the patient's best interests (*see F v. West Berkshire HA* [1989] 2 ALL ER 546). It is important to note that the relatives of an adult patient have no special status as regards his or her treatment. They cannot consent to treatment on the patient's behalf, nor can they refuse treatment. As a matter of good practice, the doctor may choose to involve the relatives in the decision-making process; relatives will often be in the best position to advise as to the treatment (if any) the patient would choose were he or she able to make a decision. As the courts have decided that a doctor is under a duty to act in the best interests of an incompetent adult, it is highly unlikely that they would preclude the disclosure of confidential information to relatives, where such a disclosure is necessary to assist in determining the treatment which would be in the patient's best interests.

The competent child
If a child under the age of 16 'reaches a sufficient understanding and intelligence to be capable of making up his own mind on the matter requiring decision', it appears that the duty of confidence is the same as that owed to a competent adult (*see* page 67).

The incompetent child
Similar former GMC guidance in relation to minors has attracted criticism, most notably from the British Medical Association (BMA). The view advanced by the then Secretary of the BMA, Dr Havard, was that in the case of an incompetent girl, the fact that she had consulted the doctor and, presumably, anything he had learned in the process of assessing her competence, must be kept secret if she so wishes.

The guidance issued by the GMC is probably an accurate statement of the law, either because a duty of confidence is not owed to the patient until he or she is competent (*see* Kennedy, 'Confidentiality, Competence and Malpractice', *Medicine in Contemporary Society: Kings College Studies 1986–7*, King Edward's Hospital Fund for London), or, as is more likely, because, whilst a duty of confidentiality can be owed to an incompetent infant patient, disclosure to a parent will not constitute a breach of confidence, if the disclosure is necessary in the interests of the infant (*see* Lord Templeman, *Gillick v. West Norfolk and Wisbech Area Health Authority* [1985] 3 ALL ER 402 at 434h).

4 Statutory disclosures

There are numerous statutory provisions which oblige a doctor to disclose certain confidential information to the appropriate authorities. This is recognized in paragraph 10 of the GMC's revised guidance, and forms the fourth exception to the obligation of confidentiality:

> Information may be disclosed in order to satisfy a specific statutory requirement, such as notification of an infectious disease or of attendance upon a person known or suspected to be addicted to a controlled drug.

The relevant statutory provisions are considered below.

(a) *Prevention and detection of crime*

The gathering of evidence by police is regulated primarily by the Police and Criminal Evidence Act 1984. Under this Act, medical records are classified as 'personal records' and therefore constitute 'excluded material' (section 11). Contrary to the view of many police officers, this prevents the police from gaining (or a judge ordering) access to a suspect's medical records under the Act (*R v. Central Criminal Court, Ex parte Brown* [1992] Queen's Bench Division (unreported)).

The only situation in which the police can compel the disclosure of medical records is in connection with offences of terrorism under the Prevention of Terrorism (Temporary Provisions) Act 1989, and then only with an inspection or search warrant or, in cases of great emergency, a written order by an officer of not less than the rank of superintendent. Although the police cannot otherwise compel the disclosure of a suspect's medical records, they may compel the disclosure of the identity of a driver suspected of committing a road traffic offence (*see* below: Identity of drivers).

The fact that the police cannot compel the disclosure of confidential information does not prevent the holder of that information from disclosing it voluntarily, provided he or she can justify the disclosure as being in the public interest (*see* page 72).

(b) *The identity of drivers*

Where the driver of a vehicle, or rider of a bicycle, is alleged to be guilty of a road traffic offence:

> . . . any other person [ie a person other than the person in possession of the vehicle] shall if required . . . [by a police officer] give such information which it is in his power to give and may lead to identification of the driver. (section 172(b), Road Traffic Act 1988)

Failure to give information in accordance with the section is an offence (section 172(4)). The fact that a doctor may have acquired such information through the doctor-patient relationship will not excuse him or her from the obligation to provide information in accordance with the section.

> In the circumstances I am driven to the conclusion that a doctor acting within his professional capacity, and carrying out his professional duties and responsibilities, is within the words 'any other person' in [the] section . . . May I say, before leaving the case, that I appreciate the concern of the responsible medical practitioner who feels that he is faced with a conflict of duty. That the defendant was conscious of a conflict and realised his duty to both society and to his patient is clear from the finding of the

justices, but he may find comfort, although the decision goes against him, from the following. First, that he has only to disclose information which may lead to identification and not other confidential matters; secondly, that the result, in my judgement, is entirely consistent with the rules that the British Medical Association have laid down. Mr Justice Boreham, *Hunter v. Mann* [1974] 1 QB 767 at 774

(c) *Terrorism*

Section 18 of the Prevention of Terrorism (Temporary Provisions) Act 1989 obliges any person who has information which he or she knows, or believes, might be of assistance:

> . . . in preventing the commission . . . of an act of terrorism connected with the affairs of Northern Ireland; or in securing the apprehension, prosecution or conviction of any other person for an offence involving the commission, preparation or instigation of such an act

to disclose that information to a constable. Failure to provide information in accordance with section 18, without reasonable excuse, is an offence punishable by imprisonment for a period of up to 10 years (section 18(2)). Ignorance of the law will not constitute a 'reasonable excuse' and, in the light of the serious threat posed to the public safety by terrorism, it is widely accepted that neither will the doctor's duty of confidence towards his or her patient.

(d) *Drug addicts*

The Misuse of Drugs (Notification of Supply to Addicts) Regulations 1973 (SI 1973/799 as amended) require that:

> . . . any doctor who attends a person who he considers, or has reasonable grounds to suspect, is addicted to any [notifiable] drug shall, within seven days of the attendance, furnish in writing to the Chief Medical Officer at the Home Office such of the following particulars with respect to that person as are known to the doctor, that is to say, the name, address, sex, date of birth and National Health Service number of that person, the date of the attendance and the name of the drug or drugs concerned. (regulation 3(1))

However, no report need be made under the regulations where:

(a) the doctor is of the opinion, formed in good faith, that the continued administration of the drug or drugs concerned is required for the purpose of treating organic disease or injury; or

(b) the particulars . . . [above] have, during the period of twelve months ending with the date of the attendance, been furnished in compliance with those provisions

   (i)   by the doctor; or

   (ii) if the doctor is a partner in or employed by a firm of general practitioners, by a doctor who is a partner in or employed by that firm; or

   (iii) if the attendance is on behalf of another doctor, whether for payment or otherwise, by that doctor; or

   (iv) if the attendance is at a hospital, by a doctor on the staff of that hospital. (regulation 3(2))

(e) *Infectious diseases*

Section 11(1) of the Public Health (Control of Diseases) Act 1984 requires that:

If a registered medical practitioner becomes aware, or suspects, that a patient whom he is attending within the district of a local authority is suffering from a notifiable disease or from food poisoning, he shall, unless he believes, and has reasonable grounds for believing, that some other registered medical practitioner has complied with this subsection with respect to the patient, forthwith send to the proper officer of the local authority for that district stating:

(a) the name, age and sex of the patient and the address of the premises where the patient is;

(b) the disease or, as the case may be, particulars of the poisoning from which the patient is, or is suspected to be, suffering and the date, or approximate date, of its onset; and

(c) if the premises are a hospital, the day on which the patient was admitted, the address of the premises from which he came there and whether or not, in the opinion of the person giving the certificate, the disease or poisoning from which the patient is, or is suspected to be, suffering was contracted in the hospital.

For the purposes of the section, a 'notifiable disease' means any of the following diseases: acute encephalitis; acute meningitis; acute poliomyelitis; anthrax; cholera; diphtheria; dysentery; food poisoning; leprosy; leptospirosis; malaria; measles; meningococcal septicaemia; mumps; ophthalmia neonatorum; paratyphoid fever; plague; rabies; relapsing fever; rubella; scarlet fever; smallpox; tetanus; tuberculosis; typhoid fever; typhus; viral haemorrhagic fever; viral hepatitis; whooping cough; and yellow fever. (Section 10, as added to by the Public Health (Infectious Diseases) Regulations 1988 (SI 1988/1546).)

Failure to comply with requirement of notification is an offence punishable by a fine of up to £200 (see section 11(4)).

(f) *Abortions*

Any registered medical practitioner who terminates a pregnancy in England or Wales is required to provide the Chief Medical Officer with notice of the termination, and any other information relating to the termination as specified in the prescribed form of notification (para 4(1), Abortion Regulations 1991 (SI 1991/449)).

Any doctor who 'wilfully contravenes or wilfully fails to comply with the requirements' of notification commits an offence punishable by a fine of up to £5000 (section 2(3)). The use of the word 'wilfully' requires that the contravention or failure be done 'deliberately and intentionally, not by accident or inadvertence' (Lord Russell, *R v. Senior* [1891] 1 QB 283 at 290).

(g) *Births*

Section 124(4) of the National Health Service Act 1977 places a statutory obligation on any person in attendance on the mother, to notify the district medical officer of the birth of any child born dead or alive after the 28th week of pregnancy. Only one notification is required. Therefore, where a midwife or the father is present at the birth, the doctor may discharge his or her statutory obligation by instructing one of them to notify the birth.

5 Disclosure in the public interest

The basis of the law's protection of confidence is that there is a public interest in preserving confidences (*see Attorney General v. Guardian Newspapers (No. 2)* [1988] 3 All ER 417). It follows that this public interest may be outweighed by some other countervailing public interest. This forms the basis of the fifth exception to be found in the GMC's revised guidance.

  Rarely, cases may arise in which disclosure in the public interest may be justified, for example a situation in which the failure to disclose appropriate information would expose the patient, or someone else, to a risk of death or serious harm. (para 10)

The vague wording of the paragraph reflects both the lack of case law and the difficulty of formulating rigid rules in the present context. Although each case has to be considered on its own merits, the recent Court of Appeal judgement in *W v. Egdell* [1990] 1 All ER 835 provides some further guidance in defining the scope of the exception.

W v. Egdell

In 1974, the plaintiff, 'W', shot and killed five people and seriously injured two others. He was later diagnosed as suffering from paranoid schizophrenia. At his trial, the Crown accepted his plea of guilty to manslaughter on the grounds of diminished responsibility and, accordingly, orders were made under sections 60 and 65 of the Mental Health Act 1959 (now sections 37 and 41 of the 1983 Act) for his indefinite detention in a secure hospital.

In 1986, Dr Ghosh, the medical officer responsible for W, formed the view that W had been cured of his illness and that, providing he remained on medication, he no longer presented a danger to the public. The doctor, therefore, recommended to the Home Secretary that W should be transferred to a regional secure unit. After W's request for a transfer was rejected by the Home Secretary, W decided to pursue an alternative avenue, namely, to make an application to a Mental Health Appeal Tribunal for a conditional discharge. To this end, W's solicitors approached Dr Egdell, a distinguished psychiatrist at the Royal Liverpool Hospital, to examine W and prepare a report for use at W's forthcoming Mental Health Tribunal hearing. However, Dr Egdell was concerned that W's longstanding interest in guns and home-made bombs had not been properly understood by the hospital and, accordingly, strongly recommended that W should not be considered for transfer.

After seeing Dr Egdell's report, W withdrew his application. On discovering that the application had been withdrawn, Dr Egdell telephoned W's solicitors to ask what would happen to his report. It was explained to him that the report would remain confidential and on their files. Dr Egdell invited W's solicitors to send a copy of the report to the acting medical director of the hospital where W was held. Following instructions from their client, the solicitors declined to do so but Dr Egdell, nevertheless, sent a copy of the report to the hospital and asked for a copy to be forwarded to the Home Secretary. W then sued Dr Egdell for breach of confidence.

Mr Justice Scott dismissed W's claim and his decision was upheld by the Court of Appeal. The Court of Appeal ruled that the case centred on the basic issue of how to balance two conflicting public interests. On the one hand, confidence should be preserved and protected by the law while, on the other, the public should be protected from potential violence.

Geoffrey Robertson QC had argued on behalf of W that the public's interest in patients being able to make full and frank disclosure to their doctors and, in particular, to their psychiatrist, without fearing that the doctor would disclose the information to others, was the dominant public interest. The Court of Appeal rejected this submission. Their lordships ruled that there was one consideration which tipped the balance decisively in favour of disclosure. Before releasing W, the responsible authority must be able to make a fully informed judgement that the risk of a repetition of his offences is so small as to be acceptable. Their lordships, therefore, fully supported the actions of Dr Egdell.

Although each case must inevitably turn on its own facts, the judgement provides two principal points of clarification.

- Firstly, the public interest defence justifies disclosure to the proper authorities, not usually to the world at large.
- Secondly, it is clear that a 'real' risk of danger to the public will be sufficient grounds to justify disclosure, even if the danger is not imminent (*see* also *R v. Crozier, Daily Telegraph*, 3 May 1990). Furthermore, it would appear from the facts of the case that a possibility of serious harm, rather than a probability, will be sufficient to constitute a 'real risk'. Cases where there is more than a negligible risk of a patient committing an offence of violence or a sexual offence or, for example, of continuing to drive when diagnosed as suffering from epilepsy, should satisfy the test. Similarly, where an HIV positive patient continues to have unprotected sexual intercourse, disclosure of his or her identity could, in the author's opinion, be justified as being in the public's interest.

However, it is unclear whether even a strong probability of a patient committing a minor offence will constitute a sufficient ground for disclosure.

Although the Court of Appeal stated in *W v. Egdell* that ultimately it is for the court to decide whether the disclosure was justified, Lord Justice Bingham stated (at page 815b) that 'In making its ruling the court will give such weight to the considered judgement of a professional man as seems in all the circumstances to be appropriate'. While the courts must ultimately be arbiters of whether a doctor's actions were justifiable, in the context of the doctor-patient relationship, the courts in practice often follow standards of accepted medical practice. (In the context of investigation, diagnosis and treatment *see Maynard v. West Midlands Regional Health Authority* [1985] 1 All ER 635; in respect of disclosure of risks *see Sidaway v. Board of Governors of Bethlem Royal Hospital* [1985] 1 All ER 643; and in relation to treatment of the incompetent adult *see F v. West Berkshire Health Authority* (above)). It is unlikely that a court will take a different approach in relation to confidentiality, and it could therefore be said that a doctor may safely disclose information, provided that he or she complies with the GMC guidance or possibly just complies with the practice of a responsible body of medical opinion.

Given the uncertainty in determining whether a disclosure may be justified as being in the public interest, in all but the clearest of cases and emergencies it is advisable to first of all apply to court for a declaration that the disclosure is lawful.

A duty to disclose?

The English courts have yet to consider whether a doctor has a legal duty to a potential victim to notify the appropriate authorities of the danger posed by a patient. Such a duty was held to exist by the Supreme Court of California in *Tarasoff v. Regents of the University of California* [1976] 551 P 2d 334.

In 1968, an overseas student at the University of California met a fellow student, Tanya Tarasoff, who he saw once a week until New Year's Eve, when they kissed. He interpreted the kiss as a symbol of betrothal and, when Tanya told him there was no significance in it, he became withdrawn and psychotic. He later consulted a psychologist to whom he confided that he was going to kill Tanya when she returned from the summer vacation. The psychologist believed the student and notified the campus police who briefly detained him, but released him when he displayed no further signs of instability. No further steps were taken either to commit the student or to warn Tanya. The following month the student went to Tanya's house and, finding her alone, murdered her.

Tanya's parents brought a civil claim against the psychologist, the campus police and the University for failing either to commit the student or to warn Tanya. Although the action was initially dismissed, an appeal judgement was given against the psychologist but not against the other defendants.

Whether the English courts would be prepared to adopt a similar approach is doubtful. Any victim would have to bring a claim in negligence. This would require the victim to establish that the doctor was under a legal duty to inform him or her of the danger or, more likely, inform the relevant authorities; that in failing to do so, the doctor behaved as no reasonable doctor would have done; and that as a consequence he or she (the victim) was harmed.

Where the threat is to the public at large, the courts will probably not consider the doctor to be under a legal duty to inform the police on the grounds that the victim is merely a member of a large unascertained class (*see Hill v. Chief Constable of West Yorkshire* [1987] 1 All ER 1173). However, where a patient makes genuine threats of serious injury to an identified person the position is less clear. In his article 'Medical confidentiality and the public interest' (*Professional Negligence*, March 1990), Michael Jones argues that it will be difficult to establish the necessary legal duty of care. Any duty, he argues, must arise from the doctor's knowledge of the danger to the victim and not from the doctor-patient relationship *per se*. However, it is well established that there is no general obligation in the law of negligence to take positive steps to confer a benefit on others by preventing harm befalling them. For example, there is no duty to shout a warning to a blind man about to walk over the edge of a cliff. By analogy, it would seem that a doctor is under no duty to give a warning concerning a dangerous patient.

6 Disclosure in connection with judicial proceedings

Various judicial and quasi-judicial bodies are empowered to order a doctor to disclose confidential information. This forms the basis of the sixth exception to be found in the GMC's revised guidance.

> Where litigation is in prospect, unless the patient has consented to disclosure or a court order has been made, information should not be disclosed by a doctor merely in response to demands from other people such as a third party's solicitor or an official of the court. A doctor may disclose such information as may be ordered by a judge or presiding officer of the court, as may a doctor summoned to assist a Coroner . . . either at an inquest or when the need for an inquest is being considered. In such circumstances the doctor should first establish the precise extent of the information which needs to be disclosed, and should not hesitate to make known any objections to the proposed disclosure, particularly when the order would involve the disclosure of confidential information about third parties.

Forms of disclosure

A court may order a doctor, or other health professional, to disclose confidential medical information, either by testifying in legal proceedings or by producing documents.

A doctor may be called to give oral testimony through examination and cross-examination. In either case, he or she may be required to disclose confidential information, without the patient's consent, in response to questions asked. The doctor must answer truthfully, unless the judge directs otherwise.

> The only profession that I know of which is given a privilege from disclosing information to a court of law is the legal profession, and then it is not the privilege of the lawyer but of his client. Take the clergyman, the banker or the medical man. None of these is entitled to refuse to answer when directed to by a judge. Let me not be mistaken. The judge will respect the confidences which each member of these honourable professions receives in the course of it, and will not direct him to answer unless not only it is relevant but also it is a proper and indeed, necessary question in the course of justice to be put and answered. A judge is the person entrusted, on behalf of the community, to weigh on the one hand the respect due to confidence in the profession and on the other hand the ultimate interest of the community in justice being done. Lord Denning, Master of the Rolls, *Attorney General v. Mulholland and Foster*, [1963] 2 QB 477 at 489–90

Refusal to answer a question when directed to do so, exposes the doctor to a charge of contempt. However, any witness who is compelled to disclose confidential information in court has absolute privilege and is protected against a later action for breach of confidence (*see Watson v. McEwan* [1905] AC 480 at 486).

As we have already seen, the courts are also empowered under the Supreme Court Act 1981 to order the disclosure of medical records for the purposes of litigation. Disclosure in such circumstances is dealt with in Section 2 of this book: 'Access and Litigation'.

The Coroner's Court

Section 21(1) of the Coroners Act 1988 provides:

In the case of an inquest into a death, the coroner may summon as a witness:

(a) any legally qualified medical practitioner appearing to him to have attended at the death of the deceased or during the last illness of the deceased; or

(b) where it appears to him that no such practitioner so attended the deceased, any legally qualified medical practitioner in actual practice in or near the place where the death occurred;

and any medical witness summoned under this section may be asked to give evidence as to how, in his opinion, the deceased came by his death.

Failure to obey a summons issued in pursuance of the section, without good and sufficient cause, is an offence punishable by a fine of up to £400 (section 21(5)).

In addition to his or her powers under section 21, the coroner also has a general power to summon witnesses. Any person who fails to appear to the summons, or refuses without lawful excuse to answer a question put to the coroner, may be fined up to £1000 or be charged with contempt (section 10(2)).

Mental Health Review Tribunal

The Mental Health Tribunals, first established under the Mental Health Act 1959, are empowered to consider the need for continuing detention under the Mental Health Act 1983. To that end, the tribunals:

. . . may take evidence on oath and subpoena any witness to appear before it or to produce documents. (Rule 14(1), Mental Health Review Tribunal Rules 1983, (SI 1983/942))

The tribunal may not, however, require any witness to disclose information or documents which he or she could not be compelled to produce at a trial (Rule 14(1)). (For a discussion of the documents which a witness cannot be compelled to produce *see* pages 38–41.)

Mental Health Act Commission

The Mental Health Act Commission was established on 1 September 1983 by the Mental Health Act Commission (Establishment and Constitution) Order 1983 (SI 1983/892) and has the task of, *inter alia*, investigating complaints made by detained patients and complaints about the exercise of compulsory powers (section 120(1) Mental Health Act 1983). To that end, the Commission is empowered by section 120(4)(b) to:

> . . . require the production of and inspect any records relating to the detention or treatment of any person who is or has been detained in a mental nursing home. (section 120(4)(b))

Inquiry ordered by Secretary of State for Health

The Secretary of State for Health is empowered by section 84 of the National Health Service Act 1977 (as amended) to order an inquiry to be held in connection with any matter arising under the Act, or under Part 1 of the National Health Service and Community Care Act 1990. Any person appointed to hold the inquiry:

(a) may by summons require any person to attend, at a time and place stated in the summons, to give evidence or to produce any documents in his custody or under his control which relate to any matter in question at the inquiry; and

(b) may take evidence on oath, and for that purpose administer oaths, or may, instead of administering an oath, require the person examined to take a solemn affirmation.

Before a person can be summoned to attend the inquiry, or to produce documents, he or she must be paid or tendered any necessary expenses (section 84(3)(a)).

Deliberate failure to give evidence, or produce documents in accordance with the section, is an offence punishable by a fine of up to £1000 and a term of imprisonment of up to six months (section 84(4)).

Health Service Commissioner

The office of the Commissioner was created in 1973 and his powers are now set out in Part V of the National Health Service Act 1977. He or she is empowered to investigate any complaint where it is alleged that either a failure in the NHS or maladministration in the Service has resulted in injustice or hardship. There are significant limitations on his remit, the most important of which prevents the Commissioner from investigating complaints concerning clinical judgement. But, so far as matters falling within his remit are concerned, he has been granted considerable powers, including the same powers as the High Court to:

> . . . require any employee, officer or other member of the relevant body concerned [ie subject to investigation] or any other person who in his opinion is able to furnish information or produce documents relevant to the investigation to furnish any such information or produce any such document.

Any person who, 'without lawful excuse', fails to comply with an order by the Commissioner may be referred to the High Court and be dealt with as though he or she had failed to comply with an order of the Court itself (National Health Act 1977, Schedule 13, paras 12–14). In order to establish a lawful excuse it is necessary to show that he or she honestly believed, and had reasonable grounds for believing, that the facts were of a certain order, and that had those facts been of that order, his or her conduct would have been lawful (*see Cambridgeshire and Isle of Ely CC v. Rust* [1972] 2 QB 426).

Employment medical advisers

The Secretary of State for Health is required to ensure that each district health authority arranges for one of its officers who is a fully registered medical practitioner to provide an employment medical adviser, when requested to do so, with:

> . . . such particulars of the school record of a person who has not yet attained the age of eighteen and such other information relating to his medical history as the adviser may reasonably require for the efficient performance of his functions. (section 60, Health and Safety at Work Act 1974)

Although the employment medical adviser does not have the power to order disclosure personally, the practical effect of the section is the same, other than to the extent that no criminal sanction is provided for failure to comply with a request for disclosure.

7 Disclosure for the purposes of teaching, research and medical audit

Paragraph 14 of the GMC's revised guidance recognizes the importance of medical teaching, research and audit:

> Medical teaching, research and medical audit necessarily involve the disclosure of information about individuals, often in the form of medical

records, for purposes other than their own health care. Where such information is used in a form which does not enable individuals to be identified, no question of breach of confidentiality will usually arise. Where the disclosure would enable one or more individuals to be identified, the patients concerned, or those who may properly give permission on their behalf, must wherever possible be made aware of that possibility and be advised that it is open to them, at any stage, to withhold their consent to disclosure.

The legal basis for such disclosures is that the patient will have consented, either expressly or indirectly, to the disclosure. However, in the absence of patient consent, for example, where the patient is comatosed, the disclosure may be justified as being in the public interest, given the long-term benefits to society. Although there is no judicial authority on the point, is is unlikely that the courts would dispute that the disclosure may be justified as being in the public interest, provided that disclosure is for an approved research or teaching programme.

Remedies for a breach of confidence or threatened breach of confidence

Injunctive relief

Interlocutory injunctions

Where the disclosure of confidential information is threatened, there may be a dispute between the parties as to whether the disclosure amounts to a breach of confidence. In such cases, the plaintiff can apply to court for an injunction restraining disclosure until the matter can be settled at a full hearing. While a so-called interlocutory injunction is a temporary measure, it is of considerable practical importance, because if the patient then fails to restrain disclosure it will usually be pointless for him to continue with his claim.

An injunction is not available as of right, but only at the discretion of the court. The principles on which the court's discretion should be exercised were laid down by Lord Diplock in *American Cyanamid Co v. Ethicon Ltd* [1975] 1 All ER 504. These detailed principles are of general application, but, in the present context, a patient should be able to obtain an interlocutory injunction provided that he or she can show that there is 'a serious issue to be tried'. In other words, the application must be shown not to be frivolous or vexatious.

Permanent injunctions

Should the patient's claim proceed to a full trial and the court rule in his or her favour, the court may grant a permanent injunction. Again, in the overwhelming majority of cases in the present context, an injunction will be granted virtually automatically. Failure to comply with the injunction may result in a fine or even imprisonment for contempt of court.

Damages

Where a breach of confidence has already occurred, an injunction will clearly be inappropriate, leaving the plaintiff with only the possibility of claiming damages.

Where the patient has suffered psychiatric or physical harm as a consequence of the breach of confidence, he or she may be able to obtain damages by bringing a claim in negligence, providing that it was foreseeable that he or she would suffer such harm as a consequence of the breach. Furthermore, it may be possible to obtain damages for personal upset if the patient has a contractual relationship with the doctor, for example, by paying for a private consultation. An implied term of such a contract will usually be that the doctor will not breach the patient's confidence. In such circumstances, a patient may be able to recover in contract damages for upset, embarrassment and distress, providing it can be shown that it was foreseeable that these were likely to result from the breach (*see Jarvis v. Swan Tours Ltd* [1973] QB 233).

However, it appears at present that a patient will ordinarily be unable to obtain damages in respect of simple upset, embarrassment or distress caused by a non-contractual breach of confidence (*see* the *Law Commission Report on Breach of Confidence* (Law Commission No. 110) at para 4.81)). Whether the law will develop so as to enable damages to be recovered in respect of a non-contractual breach of confidence is unclear. In W *v.* Egdell (page 73–4), for example, Mr Justice Scott stated that as W had suffered no tangible harm, he would not have awarded W damages had his action succeeded. The Court of Appeal, however, preferred to leave the question open.

Death of the patient

Paragraph 16 of the revised GMC guidance states:

> The fact of a patient's death does not of itself release the doctor from the obligation to maintain confidentiality. In cases where consent has not previously been given, the extent to which confidential information may properly be disclosed by a doctor after someone's death cannot be specified in absolute terms and will depend on the circumstances. These include the nature of the information disclosed, the extent to which it has already appeared in published material and the period which has elapsed since the person's death.

Any doctor who fails to maintain secrecy after a patient's death may therefore find him- or herself faced with a charge of professional misconduct. However, as a matter of law, a patient's personal representatives will be unable to sue in respect of a breach which occurred after the patient's death. This is because the information is of a personal nature rather than a 'quasi-proprietorial' nature, such as information relating to 'know-how' which may be regarded as an asset of the deceased's estate. Where, however, the breach occurs before the patient's death, then, by virtue of section 1(1) of the Law Reform (Miscellaneous Provisions) Act 1934, an action for damages may be brought by and on behalf of the deceased's estate.

Appendix

The following statutes and health circulars are reproduced with the kind permission of Her Majesty's Stationery Office and the Department of Health.

Patient Access

Data Protection Act 1984

1984 CHAPTER 35

An Act to regulate the use of automatically processed information relating to individuals and the provision of services in respect of such information.

[12th July 1984]

Be it enacted by the Queen's most Excellent Majesty, by and with the advice and consent of the Lords Spiritual and Temporal, and Commons, in this present Parliament assembled, and by the authority of the same, as follows: –

Part I: Preliminary

Definition of 'data' and related expressions

1 – (1) The following provisions shall have effect for the interpretation of this Act.

(2) 'Data' means information recorded in a form in which it can be processed by equipment operating automatically in response to instructions given for that purpose.

(3) 'Personal data' means data consisting of information which relates to a living individual who can be identified from that information (or from that and other information in the possession of the data user), including any expression of opinion about the individual but not any indication of the intentions of the data user in respect of that individual.

(4) 'Data subject' means an individual who is the subject of personal data.

(5) 'Data user' means a person who holds data, and a person 'holds' data if –

(a) the data form part of a collection of data processed or intended to be processed by or on behalf of that person as mentioned in subsection (2) above; and

(b) that person (either alone or jointly or in common with other persons) controls the contents and use of the data comprised in the collection; and

(c) the data are in the form in which they have been or are intended to be processed as mentioned in paragraph (a) above or (though not for the time being in that form) in a form into which they have been converted after being so processed and with a view to being further so processed on a subsequent occasion.

(6) A person carries on a 'computer bureau' if he provides other persons with services in respect of data, and a person provides such services if –

(a) as agent for other persons he causes data held by them to be processed as mentioned in subsection (2) above; or

(b) he allows other persons the use of equipment in his possession for the processing as mentioned in that subsection of data held by them.

(7) 'Processing', in relation to data, means amending, augmenting, deleting or re-arranging the data or extracting the information constituting the data and, in the case of personal data, means performing any of those operations by reference to the data subject.

(8) Subsection (7) above shall not be construed as applying to any operation performed only for the purpose of preparing the text of documents.

(9) 'Disclosing', in relation to data, includes disclosing information extracted from the data; and where the identification of the individual who is the subject of personal data depends partly on the information constituting the data and partly on other information in the possession of the data user, the data shall not be regarded as disclosed or transferred unless the other information is also disclosed or transferred.

The data protection principles

2 – (1) Subject to subsection (3) below, references in this Act to the data protection principles are to the principles set out in Part I of Schedule 1 to this Act; and those principles shall be interpreted in accordance with Part II of that Schedule.

(2) The first seven principles apply to personal data held by data users and the eighth applies both to such data and to personal data in respect of which services are provided by persons carrying on computer bureaux.

(3) The Secretary of State may by order modify or supplement those principles for the purpose of providing additional safeguards in relation to personal data consisting of information as to –

(a) the racial origin of the data subject;

(b) his political opinions or religious or other beliefs;

(c) his physical or mental health or his sexual life; or

(d) his criminal convictions;

and references in this Act to the data protection principles include, except where the context otherwise requires, references to any modified or additional principle having effect by virtue of an order under this subsection.

(4) An order under subsection (3) above may modify a principle either by modifying the principle itself or by modifying its interpretation; and where an order under that subsection modifies a principle or provides for an additional principle it may contain provisions for the interpretation of the modified or additional principle.

(5) An order under subsection (3) above modifying the third data protection principle may, to such extent as the Secretary of State thinks appropriate, exclude or modify in relation to that principle any exemption from the non-disclosure provisions which is contained in Part IV of this Act; and the exemptions from those provisions contained in that Part shall accordingly have effect subject to any order made by virtue of this subsection.

(6) An order under subsection (3) above may make different provision in relation to data consisting of information of different descriptions.

The Registrar and the Tribunal

3 – (1) For the purposes of this Act there shall be—

    (a) an officer known as the Data Protection Registrar (in this Act referred to as 'the Registrar'); and

    (b) a tribunal known as the Data Protection Tribunal (in this Act referred to as 'the Tribunal').

(2) The Registrar shall be appointed by Her Majesty by Letters Patent.

(3) The Tribunal shall consist of –

    (a) a chairman appointed by the Lord Chancellor after consultation with the Lord Advocate;

    (b) such number of deputy chairmen appointed as aforesaid as the Lord Chancellor may determine; and

    (c) such number of other members appointed by the Secretary of State as he may determine.

(4) The members of the Tribunal appointed under subsection (3)(a) and (b) above shall be barristers, advocates or solicitors, in each case of not less than seven years' standing.

(5) The members of the Tribunal appointed under subsection (3)(c) above shall be –

    (a) persons to represent the interests of data users; and

    (b) persons to represent the interests of data subjects.

(6) Schedule 2 to this Act shall have effect in relation to the Registrar and the Tribunal.

Part II: Registration and supervision of data users and computer bureaux

[sections 4–9 omitted]

Supervision

Enforcement notices

10 – (1) If the Registrar is satisfied that a registered person has contravened or is contravening any of the data protection principles he may serve him with a notice ('an enforcement notice') requiring him to take, within such time as is specified in the notice, such steps as are so specified for complying with the principle or principles in question.

(2) In deciding whether to serve an enforcement notice the Registrar shall consider whether the contravention has caused or is likely to cause any person damage or distress.

(3) An enforcement notice in respect of a contravention of the fifth data protection principle may require the data user –

    (a) to rectify or erase the data and any other data held by him and containing an expression of opinion which appears to the Registrar to be based on the inaccurate data; or

    (b) in the case of such data as are mentioned in subsection (2) of section 22 below; either to take the steps mentioned in paragraph (a) above or to take such steps as are specified in the notice for securing compliance with the requirements specified in that subsection and, if the Registrar thinks fit, for supplementing the data with such statement of the true facts relating to the matters dealt with by the data as the Registrar may approve.

(4) The Registrar shall not serve an enforcement notice requiring the person served with the notice to take steps for complying with paragraph (a) of the seventh data protection principle in respect of any data subject unless satisfied that the person has contravened section 21 below by failing to supply information to which the data subject is entitled and which has been duly requested in accordance with that section.

(5) An enforcement notice shall contain –

    (a) a statement of the principle or principles which the Registrar is satisfied have been or are being contravened and his reasons for reaching that conclusion; and

    (b) particulars of the rights of appeal conferred by section 13 below.

(6) Subject to subsection (7) below, the time specified in an enforcement notice for taking the steps which it requires shall not expire before the end of the period within which an appeal can be brought against the notice and, if such an appeal is brought, those steps need not be taken pending the determination or withdrawal of the appeal.

(7) If by reason of special circumstances the Registrar considers that the steps required by an enforcement notice should be taken as a matter of urgency he may include a statement to that effect in the notice; and in that event subsection (6) above shall not apply but the notice shall not require the steps to be taken before the end of the period of seven days beginning with the date on which the notice is served.

(8) The Registrar may cancel an enforcement notice by written notification to the person on whom it was served.

(9) Any person who fails to comply with an enforcement notice shall be guilty of an offence; but it shall be a defence for a person charged with an offence under this subsection to prove that he exercised all due diligence to comply with the notice in question.

De-registration notices

11 – (1) If the Registrar is satisfied that a registered person has contravened or is contravening any of the data protection principles he may –

(a) serve him with a notice ('a de-registration notice') stating that he proposes, at the expiration of such period as is specified in the notice, to remove from the register all or any of the particulars constituting the entry or any of the entries contained in the register in respect of that person; and

(b) subject to the provisions of this section, remove those particulars from the register at the expiration of that period.

(2) In deciding whether to serve a de-registration notice the Registrar shall consider whether the contravention has caused or is likely to cause any person damage or distress, and the Registrar shall not serve such a notice unless he is satisfied that compliance with the principle or principles in question cannot be adequately secured by the service of an enforcement notice.

(3) A de-registration notice shall contain –

(a) a statement of the principle or principles which the Registrar is satisfied have been or are being contravened and his reasons for reaching that conclusion and deciding that compliance cannot be adequately secured by the service of an enforcement notice; and

(b) particulars of the rights of appeal conferred by section 13 below.

(4) Subject to subsection (5) below, the period specified in a de-registration notice pursuant to subsection (1)(a) above shall not expire

before the end of the period within which an appeal can be brought against the notice and, if such an appeal is brought, the particulars shall not be removed pending the determination or withdrawal of the appeal.

(5) If by reason of special circumstances the Registrar considers that any particulars should be removed from the register as a matter of urgency he may include a statement to that effect in the de-registration notice; and in that event subsection (4) above shall not apply but the particulars shall not be removed before the end of the period of seven days beginning with the date on which the notice is served.

(6) The Registrar may cancel a de-registration notice by written notification to the person on whom it was served.

(7) References in this section to removing any particulars include references to restricting any description which forms part of any particulars.

[Sections 12 – 19 omitted]

Liability of directors, etc

20 – (1) Where an offence under this Act has been committed by a body corporate and is proved to have been committed with the consent or connivance of or to be attributable to any neglect on the part of any director, manager, secretary or similar officer of the body corporate or any person who was purporting to act in any such capacity, he as well as the body corporate shall be guilty of that offence and be liable to be proceeded against and punished accordingly.

(2) Where the affairs of a body corporate are managed by its members subsection (1) above shall apply in relation to the acts and defaults of a member in connection with his functions of management as if he were a director of the body corporate.

Part III: Rights of data subjects

Right of access to personal data

21 – (1) Subject to the provisions of this section, an individual shall be entitled –

- (a) to be informed by any data user whether the data held by him include personal data of which that individual is the data subject; and
- (b) to be supplied by any data user with a copy of the information constituting any such personal data held by him;

and where any of the information referred to in paragraph (b) above is expressed in terms which are not intelligible without explanation the information shall be accompanied by an explanation of those terms.

(2) A data user shall not be obliged to supply any information under subsection (1) above except in response to a request in writing and on payment of such fee (not exceeding the prescribed maximum) as he may require; but a request for information under both paragraphs of that subsection shall be treated as a single request and a request for information under paragraph (a) shall, in the absence of any indication to the contrary, be treated as extending also to information under paragraph (b).

(3) In the case of a data user having separate entries in the register in respect of data held for different purposes a separate request must be made and a separate fee paid under this section in respect of the data to which each entry relates.

(4) A data user shall not be obliged to comply with a request under this section –

(a) unless he is supplied with such information as he may reasonably require in order to satisfy himself as to the identity of the person making the request and to locate the information which he seeks; and

(b) if he cannot comply with the request without disclosing information relating to another individual who can be identified from that information, unless he is satisfied that the other individual has consented to the disclosure of the information to the person making the request.

(5) In paragraph (b) of subsection (4) above the reference to information relating to another individual includes a reference to information identifying that individual as the source of the information sought by the request; and that paragraph shall not be construed as excusing a data user from supplying so much of the information sought by the request as can be supplied without disclosing the identity of the other individual concerned, whether by the omission of names or other identifying particulars or otherwise.

(6) A data user shall comply with a request under this section within forty days of receiving the request or, if later, receiving the information referred to in paragraph (a) of subsection (4) above and, in a case where it is required, the consent referred to in paragraph (b) of that subsection.

(7) The information to be supplied pursuant to a request under this section shall be supplied by reference to the data in question at the time when the request is received except that it may take account of any amendment or deletion made between that time and the time when the information is supplied, being an amendment or deletion that would have been made regardless of the receipt of the request.

(8) If a court is satisfied on the application of any person who has made a request under the foregoing provisions of this section that the data user in question has failed to comply with the request in contravention of those provisions, the court may order him to comply with the request; but a court shall not make an order under this subsection if it considers that it would in all the circumstances be unreasonable to do so, whether because of the frequency with which the applicant has made requests to the data user under those provisions or for any other reason.

(9) The Secretary of State may by order provide for enabling a request under this section to be made on behalf of any individual who is incapable by reason of mental disorder of managing his own affairs.

Compensation for inaccuracy

22 – (1) An individual who is the subject of personal data held by a data user and who suffers damage by reason of the inaccuracy of the data shall be entitled to compensation from the data user for that damage and for any distress which the individual has suffered by reason of the inaccuracy.

(2) In the case of data which accurately record information received or obtained by the data user from the data subject or a third party, subsection (1) above does not apply if the following requirements have been complied with –

    (a) the data indicate that the information was received or obtained as aforesaid or the information has not been extracted from the data except in a form which includes an indication to that effect; and

    (b) if the data subject has notified the data user that he regards the information as incorrect or misleading, an indication to that effect has been included in the data or the information has not been extracted from the data except in a form which includes an indication to that effect.

(3) In proceedings brought against any person by virtue of this section it shall be a defence to prove that he had taken such care as in all the circumstances was reasonably required to ensure the accuracy of the data at the material time.

(4) Data are inaccurate for the purposes of this section if incorrect or misleading as to any matter of fact.

Compensation for loss or unauthorised disclosure

23 – (1) An individual who is the subject of personal data held by a data user or in respect of which services are provided by a person carrying on a computer bureau and who suffers damage by reason of –

    (a) the loss of the data;

    (b) the destruction of the data without the authority of the data user or, as the case may be, of the person carrying on the bureau; or

(c) subject to subsection (2) below, the disclosure of the data, or access having been obtained to the data, without such authority as aforesaid,

shall be entitled to compensation from the data user, or, as the case may be, the person carrying on the bureau for that damage and for any distress which the individual has suffered by reason of the loss, destruction, disclosure or access.

(2) In the case of a registered data user, subsection (1)(c) above does not apply to disclosure to, or access by, any person falling within a description specified pursuant to section 4(3)(d) above in an entry in the register relating to that data user.

(3) In proceedings brought against any person by virtue of this section it shall be a defence to prove that he had taken such care as in all the circumstances was reasonably required to prevent the loss, destruction, disclosure or access in question.

Rectification and erasure

24 – (1) If a court is satisfied on the application of a data subject that personal data held by a data user of which the applicant is the subject are inaccurate within the meaning of section 22 above, the court may order the rectification or erasure of the data and of any data held by the data user and containing an expression of opinion which appears to the court to be based on the inaccurate data.

(2) Subsection (1) above applies whether or not the data accurately record information received or obtained by the data user from the data subject or a third party but where the data accurately record such information, then –

(a) if the requirements mentioned in section 22(2) above have been complied with, the court may, instead of making an order under subsection (1) above, make an order requiring the data to be supplemented by such statement of the true facts relating to the matters dealt with by the data as the court may approve; and

(b) if all or any of those requirements have not been complied with, the court may, instead of making an order under that subsection, make such order as it thinks fit for securing compliance with those requirements with or without a further order requiring the data to be supplemented by such a statement as is mentioned in paragraph (a) above.

(3) If a court is satisfied on the application of a data subject –

(a) that he has suffered damage by reason of the disclosure of personal data, or of access having been obtained to personal data, in circumstances entitling him to compensation under section 23 above; and

(b) that there is a substantial risk of further disclosure of or access to the data without such authority as is mentioned in that section.

the court may order the erasure of the data; but, in the case of data in respect of which services were being provided by a person carrying on a computer bureau, the court shall not make such an order unless such steps as are reasonably practicable have been taken for notifying the person for whom those services were provided and giving him an opportunity to be heard.

Jurisdiction and procedure

25 – (1) The jurisdiction conferred by sections 21 and 24 above shall be exercisable by the High Court or a county court or, in Scotland, by the Court of Session or the sheriff.

(2) For the purpose of determining any question whether an applicant under subsection (8) of section 21 above is entitled to the information which he seeks (including any question whether any relevant data are exempt from that section by virtue of Part IV of this Act) a court may require the information constituting any data held by the data user to be made available for its own inspection but shall not, pending the determination of that question in the applicant's favour, require the information sought by the applicant to be disclosed to him or his representatives whether by discovery (or, in Scotland, recovery) or otherwise.

Part IV: Exemptions

Preliminary

26 – (1) References in any provision of Part II or III of this Act to personal data do not include references to data which by virtue of this Part of this Act are exempt from that provision.

(2) In this Part of this Act 'the subject access provisions' means –

(a) section 21 above; and
(b) any provision of Part II of this Act conferring a power on the Registrar to the extent to which it is exercisable by reference to paragraph (a) of the seventh data protection principle.

(3) In this Part of this Act 'the non-disclosure provisions' means –

(a) sections 5(2)(d) and 15 above; and
(b) any provision of Part II of this Act conferring a power on the Registrar to the extent to which it is exercisable by reference to any data protection principle inconsistent with the disclosure in question.

(4) Except as provided by this Part of this Act the subject access provisions shall apply notwithstanding any enactment or rule of law prohibiting or restricting the disclosure, or authorising the withholding, of information.

[Sections 27 & 28 omitted]

Health and social work

29 – (1) The Secretary of State may by order exempt from the subject access provisions, or modify those provisions in relation to, personal data consisting of information as to the physical or mental health of the data subject.

(2) The Secretary of State may by order exempt from the subject access provisions, or modify those provisions in relation to, personal data of such other descriptions as may be specified in the order, being information –

- (a) held by government departments or local authorities or by voluntary organisations or other bodies designated by or under the order; and
- (b) appearing to him to be held for, or acquired in the course of, carrying out social work in relation to the data subject or other individuals;

but the Secretary of State shall not under this subsection confer any exemption or make any modification except so far as he considers that the application to the data of those provisions (or of those provisions without modification) would be likely to prejudice the carrying out of social work.

(3) An order under this section may make different provision in relation to data consisting of information of different descriptions.

[Sections 30 & 31(1) omitted]

31 – (2) Personal data are exempt from the subject access provisions if the data consist of information in respect of which a claim to legal professional privilege (or, in Scotland, to confidentiality as between client and professional legal adviser) could be maintained in legal proceedings.

[Sections 32–33(5) omitted]

33 – (6) Personal data held only for –

- (a) preparing statistics; or
- (b) carrying out research,

are exempt from the subject access provisions; but it shall be a condition of that exemption that the data are not used or disclosed for any other purpose and that the resulting statistics or the results of the research are not made available in a form which identifies the data subjects or any of them.

Other exemptions

34 – (1) Personal data held by any person are exempt from the provisions of Part II of this Act and of sections 21 to 24 above if the data consist of information which that person is required by or under any enactment to make available to the public, whether by publishing it, making it available for inspection or otherwise and whether gratuitously or on payment of a fee.

(2) The Secretary of State may by order exempt from the subject access provisions personal data consisting of information the disclosure of which is prohibited or restricted by or under any enactment if he considers that the prohibition or restriction ought to prevail over those provisions in the interests of the data subject or of any other individual.

[Section 34(3) omitted]

(4) Personal data are exempt from the subject access provisions if the data are kept only for the purpose of replacing other data in the event of the latter being lost, destroyed or impaired.

(5) Personal data are exempt from the non-disclosure provisions in any case in which the disclosure is –

(a) required by or under any enactment, by any rule of law or by the order of a court; or

(b) made for the purpose of obtaining legal advice or for the purposes of, or in the course of, legal proceedings in which the person making the disclosure is a party or a witness.

(6) Personal data are exempt from the non-disclosure provisions in any case in which –

(a) the disclosure is to the data subject or a person acting on his behalf; or

(b) the data subject or any such person has requested or consented to the particular disclosure in question; or

(c) the disclosure is by a data user or a person carrying on a computer bureau to his servant or agent for the purpose of enabling the servant or agent to perform his functions as such; or

(d) the person making the disclosure has reasonable grounds for believing that the disclosure falls within any of the foregoing paragraphs of this subsection.

(7) Section 4(3)(d) above does not apply to any disclosure falling within paragraph (a), (b) or (c) of subsection (6) above; and that subsection shall apply to the restriction on disclosure in section 33(6) above as it applies to the non-disclosure provisions.

(8) Personal data exempt from the non-disclosure provisions in any case in which the disclosure is urgently required for preventing injury or other damage to the health of any person or persons; and in proceedings against any person for contravening a provision mentioned in section 26(3)(a) above it shall be a defence to prove that he had reasonable grounds for believing that the disclosure in question was urgently required for that purpose.

(9) A person need not comply with a notice, request or order under the subject access provisions if compliance would expose him to proceedings for any offence other than an offence under this Act; and information disclosed by any person in compliance with such a notice, request or order shall not be admissible against him in proceedings for an offence under this Act.

[Section 35 omitted]

Part V: General

General duties of Registrar

36 – (1) It shall be the duty of the Registrar so to perform his functions under this Act as to promote the observance of the data protection principles by data users and persons carrying on computer bureaux.

(2) The Registrar may consider any complaint that any of the data protection principles or any provision of this Act has been or is being contravened and shall do so if the complaint appears to him to raise a matter of substance and to have been made without undue delay by a person directly affected; and where the Registrar considers any such complaint he shall notify the complainant of the result of his consideration and of any action which he proposes to take.

(3) The Registrar shall arrange for the dissemination in such form and manner as he considers appropriate of such information as it may appear to him expedient to give to the public about the operation of this Act and other matters within the scope of his functions under this Act and may give advice to any person as to any of those matters.

[Sections 36(4)–40 omitted]

General interpretation

41 In addition to the provisions of sections 1 and 2 above, the following provisions shall have effect for the interpretation of this Act –

'business' includes any trade or profession;

'data equipment' means equipment for the automatic processing of data or for recording information so that it can be automatically processed;

'data material' means any document or other material used in connection with data equipment;

'a de-registration notice' means a notice under section 11 above;

'enactment' includes an enactment passed after this Act;

'an enforcement notice' means a notice under section 10 above;

'the European Convention' means the Convention for the Protection of Individuals with regard to Automatic Processing of Personal Data which was opened for signature on 28th January 1981;

'government department' includes a Northern Ireland department and any body or authority exercising statutory functions on behalf of the Crown;

'prescribed' means prescribed by regulations made by the Secretary of State;

'the Registrar' means the Data Protection Registrar;

'the register', except where the reference is to the register of companies, means the register maintained under section 4 above and (except where the reference is to a registered company, to the registered office of a company or to registered post) references to registration shall be construed accordingly;

'registered company' means a company registered under the enactments relating to companies for the time being in force in any part of the United Kingdom;

'a transfer prohibition notice' means a notice under section 12 above;

'the Tribunal' means the Data Protection Tribunal.

SCHEDULES

SCHEDULE 1: THE DATA PROTECTION PRINCIPLES (Section 2(1))

Part I: The principles

Personal data held by data users

1 The information to be contained in personal data shall be obtained, and personal data shall be processed, fairly and lawfully.

2 Personal data shall be held only for one or more specified and lawful purposes.

3 Personal data held for any purpose or purposes shall not be used or disclosed in any manner incompatible with that purpose or those purposes.

4 Personal data held for any purpose or purposes shall be adequate, relevant and not excessive in relation to that purpose or those purposes.

5 Personal data shall be accurate and, where necessary, kept up to date.

6 Personal data held for any purpose or purposes shall not be kept for longer than is necessary for that purpose or those purposes.

7 An individual shall be entitled –
   (a) at reasonable intervals and without undue delay or expense –
      (i) to be informed by any data user whether he holds personal data of which that individual is the subject; and
      (ii) to access to any such data held by a data user; and
   (b) where appropriate, to have such data corrected or erased.

Personal data held by data users or in respect of which services are provided by persons carrying on computer bureaux

8 Appropriate security measures shall be taken against unauthorised access to, or alteration, disclosure or destruction of, personal data and against accidental loss or destruction of personal data.

Part II: Interpretation

The first principle

1 – (1) Subject to sub-paragraph (2) below, in determining whether information was obtained fairly regard shall be had to the method by which it was obtained, including in particular whether any person from whom it was obtained was deceived or misled as to the purpose or purposes for which it is to be held, used or disclosed.

(2) Information shall in any event be treated as obtained fairly if it is obtained from a person who –

(a) is authorised by or under an enactment to supply it; or
(b) is required to supply it by or under any enactment or by any convention or other instrument imposing an international obligation on the United Kingdom;

and in determining whether information was obtained fairly there shall be disregarded any disclosure of the information which is authorised or required by or under any enactment or required by any such convention or other instrument as aforesaid.

The second principle

2 Personal data shall not be treated as held for a specified purpose unless that purpose is described in particulars registered under this Act in relation to the data.

The third principle

3 Personal data shall not be treated as used or disclosed in contravention of this principle unless –

(a) used otherwise than for a purpose of a description registered under this Act in relation to the data; or
(b) disclosed otherwise than to a person of a description so registered.

The fifth principle

4 Any question whether or not personal data are accurate shall be determined as for the purposes of section 22 of this Act but, in the case of such data as are mentioned in subsection (2) of that section, this principle shall not be regarded as having been contravened by reason of any inaccuracy in the information there mentioned if the requirements specified in that subsection have been complied with.

The seventh principle

5 – (1) Paragraph (a) of this principle shall not be construed as conferring any rights inconsistent with section 21 of this Act.

(2) In determining whether access to personal data is sought at reasonable intervals regard shall be had to the nature of the data, the purpose for which the data are held and the frequency with which the data are altered.

(3) The correction or erasure of personal data is appropriate only where necessary for ensuring compliance with the other data protection principles.

The eighth principle

6 Regard shall be had –

(a) to the nature of the personal data and the harm that would result from such access, alteration, disclosure, loss or destruction as are mentioned in this principle; and

(b) to the place where the personal data are stored, to security measures programmed into the relevant equipment and to measures taken for ensuring the reliability of staff having access to the data.

Use for historical, statistical or research purposes

7 Where personal data are held for historical, statistical or research purposes and not used in such a way that damage or distress is, or is likely to be, caused to any data subject –

(a) the information contained in the data shall not be regarded for the purposes of the first principle as obtained unfairly by reason only that its use for any such purpose was not disclosed when it was obtained; and

(b) the data may, notwithstanding the sixth principle, be kept indefinitely.

Data Protection (Subject Access Modification) (Health) Order 1987

Made	*9th November 1987*
Coming into force	*11th November 1987*

Whereas a draft of this Order has been laid before and approved by a resolution of each House of Parliament:

Now, therefore, in exercise of the powers conferred upon me by section 29(1) and (3) of the Data Protection Act 1984 (**a**) and after consultation with the Data Protection Registrar in accordance with section 40(3) of that Act, I hereby make the following Order:

1 This Order may be cited as the Data Protection (Subject Access Modification) (Health) Order 1987 and shall come into force on 11th November 1987.

2 In this Order –

'the Act' means the Data Protection Act 1984;

'care' includes examination, investigation and diagnosis;

'dental practitioner' and 'medical practitioner' mean, respectively, a person registered under the Dentists Act 1984(**b**) and the Medical Act 1983(**c**);

'health authority' has the same meaning as in section 128(1) of the National Health Service Act 1977(**d**);

'Health Board' has the same meaning as in section 108(1) of the National Health Service (Scotland) Act 1978(**e**);

'Health and Social Services Board' has the same meaning as in Article 16 of the Health and Personal Social Services (Northern Ireland) Order 1972(**f**);

(**a**) 1984 c. 35.
(**b**) 1984 c. 24.
(**c**) 1983 c. 54.
(**d**) 1977 c. 49. This definition was amended by Schedule 3 to 1984 c. 48.
(**e**) 1978 c. 29.
(**f**) S.I. 1972/1265 (N.I. 14.).

'health professional' means any person listed in the Schedule to this Order; and

'the subject access provisions' has the meaning which it has for the purposes of Part IV of the Act.

3 – (1) This Order applies to personal data consisting of information as to the physical or mental health of the data subject if –

(a) the data are held by a health professional; or

(b) the data are held by a person other than a health professional but the information constituting the data was first recorded by or on behalf of a health professional.

(2) This Order is without prejudice to any exemption from the subject access provisions contained in any provision of the Act or of any Order made under the Act.

4 – (1) The subject access provisions shall not have effect in relation to any personal data to which this Order applies in any case where either of the requirements specified in paragraph (2) below is satisfied with respect to the information constituting the data and the obligations contained in paragraph (5) below are complied with by the data user.

(2) The requirements referred to in paragraph (1) above are that the application of the subject access provisions –

(a) would be likely to cause serious harm to the physical or mental health of the data subject; or

(b) would be likely to disclose to the data subject the identity of another individual (who has not consented to the disclosure of the information) either as a person to whom the information or part of it relates or as the source of the information or enable that identity to be deduced by the data subject either from the information itself or from a combination of that information and other information which the data subject has or is likely to have.

(3) Paragraph (2) above shall not be construed as excusing a data user –

(a) from supplying the information sought by the request for subject access where the only individual whose identity is likely to be disclosed or deduced as mentioned in sub-paragraph (b) thereof is a health professional who has been involved in the care of the data subject and the information relates to him or he supplied the information in his capacity as a health professional; or

(b) from supplying so much of the information sought by the request as can be supplied without causing serious harm as mentioned in sub-paragraph (a) thereof or enabling the identity of another individual to be disclosed or deduced as mentioned in sub-paragraph *(b)* thereof, whether by the omission of names or other particulars or otherwise.

(4) In relation to data to which this Order applies, section 21 of the Act shall have effect as if subsections (4)*(b)* and (5) were omitted and as if the reference in subsection (6) to the consent referred to in the said section 21(4)*(b)* were a reference to the consent referred to in paragraph (2)*(b)* above.

(5) A data user who is not a health professional shall not supply information constituting data to which this Order applies in response to a request under section 21 and shall not withhold any such information on the ground that one of the requirements specified in paragraph (2) above is satisfied with respect to the information unless the data user has first consulted the person who appears to the data user to be the appropriate health professional on the question whether either or both of those requirements is or are so satisfied.

(6) In paragraph (5) above 'the appropriate health professional' means –

- *(a)* the medical practitioner or dental practitioner who is currently or was most recently responsible for the clinical care of the data subject in connection with the matters to which the information which is the subject of the request relates; or
- *(b)* where there is more than one such practitioner, the practitioner who is the most suitable to advise on the matters to which the information which is the subject of the request relates; or
- *(c)* where there is no practitioner available falling within sub-paragraph *(a)* or *(b)* above, a health professional who has the necessary experience and qualifications to advise on the matters to which the information which is the subject of the request relates.

(7) Section 21(8) of the Act shall have effect, in relation to data to which this Order applies, as if the reference therein to a contravention of the foregoing provisions of that section included a reference to a contravention of the provisions contained in this Article.

Home Office   *Douglas Hurd*
9th November 1987   One of Her Majesty's
                                       Principal Secretaries of State

Data Protection Act 1984: Modified Access to Personal Health Information (HC(87)14)

DEPARTMENT OF HEALTH AND SOCIAL SECURITY: HEALTH SERVICE MANAGEMENT CIRCULAR

To:

Regional Health Authorities
District Health Authorities
Special Health Authorities for the London Postgraduate
   Teaching Hospitals
Family Practitioner Committees
} for action

Mental Health Act Commission
Community Health Councils
} for information

September 1987

Unless otherwise notified, this circular but not the Order to which it refers will cease to be valid on 10 November 1992.*

Summary

1 This circular advises on the terms of an Order which the Secretary of State proposes to lay before Parliament and which, subject to Parliament's wishes will come into effect on 11 November 1987. A copy of the proposed terms of the Order together with guidelines on the procedures for implementing the provisions of the Order are enclosed.

---

* The validity of the guidance contained in HC(87)14 is extended, by virtue of HC(89)29, until 31 October 1994.

Caveat

2 This circular must not be read as an indication of Parliament's approval of the Order. The Order may be amended before it is laid and once it has been laid it will be subject to affirmative resolution in both Houses of Parliament. This circular and its enclosures are being made available now so that data users can undertake preliminary planning arrangements. Whether it will be necessary to implement or alter these arrangements will depend on the wishes of Parliament.

Background

3 The Data Protection Act 1984 gives new rights to people about whom information is recorded on computer. They may find out information about themselves, challenge it if appropriate and claim compensation in certain circumstances.

4 From 11 November 1987 any one will be entitled, on making a written request and paying a fee, to be supplied by any 'data user' with a copy of any personal data held about him or her. The information need not necessarily be supplied as a printout. The data user may choose to write or type the information to be supplied with any accompanying explanation. A request for 'subject access' must be responded to within 40 days. If it is not, the applicant (in legal terms, the 'data subject') is entitled to complain to the Data Protection Registrar.

5 Section 29(1) of the Data Protection Act 1984 allows the Secretary of State to exempt from subject access personal data about the 'data subject's' physical or mental health or to modify the subject access provisions in relation to this type of personal data.

6 The Secretary of State has agreed that an Order should be made to modify the provisions of subject access relating to personal health data. The proposed terms of the Order are at Annex A.* This should be read in conjunction with the draft procedural guidelines which are enclosed at Annex B.

Modified subject access to personal health data

7 The Order allows access to data relating to the physical or mental health of the data subject to be modified to enable a data user to withhold

---

*Annex A reproduces the terms of the Data Protection (Subject Access Modification) (Health) Order 1987 – *see* pages 104–6.

data which is likely to cause serious harm to the physical or mental health of the data subject or another person, and data which would lead to identification of another individual other than a 'health professional'** who has been involved in the care of the data subject.

8 The general assumption is that data subjects will normally be provided with access to personal health information held about them on computers and modification of that access will only be allowed in the limited circumstances described in paragraph 7 above.

9 A data user who is not a health professional is required to consult the appropriate health professional as defined in the Order before providing or withholding access. In the absence of a response to a request for advice on whether information should be withheld, the data user is obliged to provide access to the applicant.

10 The data to which the Order applies is defined in article 3 of the Order.

Procedures

11 The Act does not prescribe the use of a standard request form. A form would however be useful in advising the data subject about the access arrangements, to ensure that all the information which is administratively necessary is provided by the data subject and to obtain the consent of the data subject to the report being copied to his general practitioner.

12 The appeals procedure for personal health information will be the same as that set out in the Data Protection Act 1984. The Data Protection Registrar will have the benefit of medical advice.

ANNEX B: Guidelines for a modified access procedure for computerised personal health information

Administration

1 Each subject access application must be examined to confirm its validity and that the prescribed fee has been paid. (The statutory time limit for providing access commences from the date when the application has been accepted as valid and the fee has been received. Receipt of a valid application should be logged.)

**The term 'health professional' means any person specified in the schedule to the Order.

[Now *see* HC(87)26 at para 3, reproduced on page 118]

2 The application may be made by a data subject, by a person authorised by the data subject, [by a person in *loco parentis*], by a person authorised to act on behalf of the data subject, or by a person having a power of attorney. Where the applicant is not the data subject, the applicant should receive only the information which would otherwise have been made available to the data subject.

3 If the application is defective the applicant must be advised.

4 If the application is valid and a computer record is held in respect of the data subject the data user should obtain a copy of the printout.

5 The data user should confirm whether the record(s) include(s) personal health data. (Personal health data means *any* personal information relating to the physical or mental health of any person from which that person can be identified and will include all information collected from the patient or other sources, or created or added to by the data user. Details of birth, address etc within a health provision context are personal health data.)

6 If personal health data is not involved the application should be processed administratively.

7 If the record includes personal health data but does not include all the clinical notes, the manual records should be obtained so that the health professionals (HPs) responsible for the clinical care of the subject can be identified. These records, or copies of them, may have to be retrieved from other locations.

The data user's procedures must ensure that confidentiality of patients' records are fully protected. If subject access and other aspects of data protection are co-ordinated separately, reference to and liaison with medical records administrators will be necessary.

8 The data user should identify the person who appears to be the appropriate health professional to be consulted about whether personal health information should be withheld (the lead HP) and should not proceed with the data subject's application for access without doing so.

9 A lay data user should always send the papers (validated access request, computer printout and manual records) to the lead HP. The inclusion of the manual records is to help the lead HP to identify which other health professionals should be consulted and to help him decide whether access to the computerised data should be modified.

Consultation with health professionals

Note. In all cases the data user should seek the advice of the medical or dental practitioner who has had clinical responsibility for the data subject and this practitioner should seek the views of other health professionals who have had a significant input to the data subject's care. In the circumstances where such a practitioner is not available or has not had clinical responsibility for the data subject, the data user should seek the advice of the health professional who seems most appropriate to advise on the subject matter of the request, eg a nurse, health visitor or a clinical psychologist.

10 The lead HP's actions commence with the receipt of the papers from a lay data user or, if he himself is the data user, from the time he has collected all the papers together.

11 The lead HP should examine the papers to identify any other HPs who have first recorded data or on whose behalf data has first been recorded, who have had a significant input to the data subject's care and whose advice on whether to withhold data may be needed.

12 The lead HP may wish to defer to another HP who has been clinically responsible for a more significant aspect of the subject's care and who will then be regarded as the lead HP.

13 The other HPs should be consulted if reasonably practicable. This may involve circulating copies of the papers to other locations. The original record should be available in an emergency.

14 Each HP consulted should familiarise himself with the Order under Section 29(1) of the Act and indicate:

(i) the computerised data which should not be disclosed because it is likely to cause serious harm to the physical or mental health of the data subject or another person;
(ii) the computerised data which should not be disclosed because it is likely to lead to the identification of another individual other than a health professional who has been involved in the care of the data subject.

The papers should be returned to the lead HP.

15 The lead HP should ensure that other HPs have had the opportunity to make their views known.

16 The lead HP should take account of the views received from other HPs and he should advise what computerised data is likely to cause serious harm and what information relating to other individuals should be withheld. He should bear in mind what the data subject already knows of his manual record and that **only information held on computer is required to be disclosed** under the terms of the Data Protection Act.

17 The lead HP should prepare a report of *all* the computerised information which can be released to the applicant taking account of the advice of other HP(s) ensuring that it is in terms which are intelligible to the applicant. This does not entail describing the significance of a particular differential diagnosis or of a particular pathological value.

18 The lead HP should also prepare a separate summary indicating the various points which may have to be explained to the data applicant and who is the most appropriate HP to give an explanation and to provide any counselling that may be considered necessary. A further summary should indicate the data that has been withheld and the reasons for withholding it. This summary should be held in the notes for future reference and not be given to the data subject.

19 The papers should be returned to the data user, if the HP is not himself the data user.

Arrangements for disclosure

Note. The fact that information has been withheld could be as harmful to data subjects as the information itself. Data users are therefore advised not to inform only those applicants from whom data has been withheld but to preface all reports with a standard disclaimer, eg:

'This report consists of all the computerised information which [I am] [this authority is] obliged to provide under the terms of the Data Protection Act 1984 as modified by the Data (Subject Access Modification) (Health) Order 1987.'

If the Data Subject enquires whether information has been withheld, the data user may offer an explanation of the terms of the Section 29(1) Order. The data user is not obliged to disclose whether information has been withheld or not. If a data user who is not a health professional discloses the fact that information has been withheld, the lead health professional must be notified as soon as possible.

20 The data user should ensure that the lead HP's report and summaries are clearly understood and recorded and should normally abide by the lead HP's advice.

21 If the lead HP has advised that no explanation or counselling is necessary, the data user should forward the report to the data applicant, advise him where he may seek further explanation if he wishes, and where the data subject has consented, send a copy of the report to the data subject's GP.

22 If the lead HP has advised that an explanation and/or counselling is necessary, the data user should arrange an appointment for the appropriate HP to see the data subject and/or applicant.

23 When the appointment has been confirmed and prior to the consultation, all relevant papers, including the report and summaries should be sent to the appropriate HP.

24 At the interview the HP should explain the report and provide any necessary counselling. He should give the report to the data applicant and advise him where he might seek further advice or help if this is appropriate.

Disposal

25 After the meeting the HP should return the papers to the data user and, if the data subject has consented, send a copy of the report to the data subject's GP.

26 The data user should record the details of all instances in which access has been modified either on the grounds that it is likely to cause serious harm or lead to the identification of another individual.

27 All records should be returned to the appropriate location.

Flowchart for procedures

The actions set out above are intended to help health authorities implement the requirements of the modified access to personal health information provisions under the Data Protection Act. Authorities may wish to adapt the arrangements, to meet their own local circumstances or to supplement the guidelines with further instructions.

A flowchart summarising these procedures follows on pages 115–16. Activities are distinguished in accordance with the symbol key, on page 114, between actions taken by the data user (or someone acting administratively on his behalf) and actions by the health professional who will advise the data user about the withholding of data.

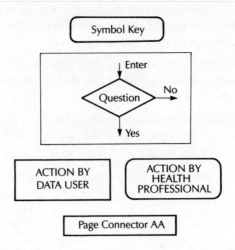

[N.B. The following flowchart contains the amendments made by HC(87)26.]

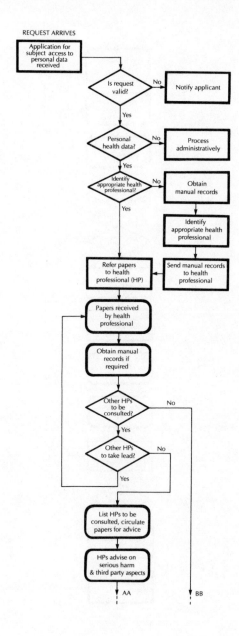

Continued on page 116

Contd.

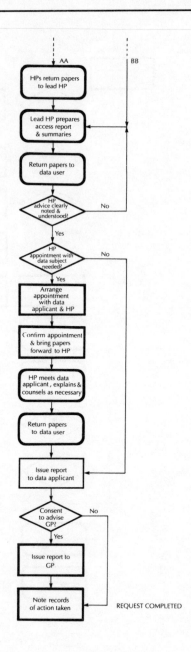

Data Protection Act 1984: Modified Access to Personal Health Information (HC(87)26) [as amended by HC(89)29]

DEPARTMENT OF HEALTH AND SOCIAL SECURITY: HEALTH SERVICE MANAGEMENT CIRCULAR

To:

Regional Health Authorities District Health Authorities Special Health Authorities for the London Postgraduate Teaching Hospitals Family Practitioner Committees Dental Estimates Board Prescription Pricing Authority	for action
Mental Health Act Commission Community Health Councils	for information

November 1987

Unless otherwise notified, this circular but not the Order to which it refers will cease to be valid on 10 November 1992.*

Summary

1 Circular HC(87)14 advised on the terms of an Order which is expected to come into effect on 11 November 1987. This circular describes certain amendments to the draft Order and guidelines which accompanied HC(87)14 and gives guidance as to the rights of children and parents under the Act.

---

*The validity of the guidance contained in HC(87)26 is extended, by virtue of HC(89)29, until 31 October 1994.

The Order

2 The draft Order proposed, by virtue of section 29(1) of the Data Protection Act 1984, that data users may withhold or modify information where disclosure 'would be likely to cause serious harm to the physical or mental health of the data subject *or any other person*'. The Data Protection Registrar and the Home Office have taken the view that the words 'or any other person' cannot be supported in law as they run counter to Recommendation R(81)1 of the Council of Europe regulations for Automated Medical Data Banks. The words 'or any other person' have therefore been deleted from the draft Order and are not to form the basis or criteria upon which to withhold or modify the disclosure of data under the Act.

The fee

3 The guidelines which accompanied HC(87)14 as appendix B suggested in paragraph 1 that the statutory time limit for providing access commences from the date when the application has been accepted as valid and the fee has been paid. This recommendation was based on the Data Protection Registrar's published advice that 'if a data user charges a fee, the individual should pay it when making the request'. The Data Protection Registrar has taken further advice on this interpretation and now holds the view that payment of the fee is not an essential requirement to fulfil before the 40 day limit commences. The Data Protection Registrar supports the practice of *requesting* payment of the fee with the application and a request for the fee may therefore be incorporated within the application forms. Data users are asked to note that a data response to a subject access request does not have to be supplied until a fee has been paid but that the 40 day period within which data users must comply starts when a valid written application has been received whether or not the fee is paid at that time.

Children

4 Paragraph 16 of HC(87)14 promised policy guidance on the position of children and the rights of parents under the Act. Advice is given in appendix 1 to this circular.

Flowchart

5 A revised flowchart is enclosed at appendix 2. This makes clear that data users do not have to scrutinise manual records if local procedures

otherwise enable the appropriate health professional to be identified without this scrutiny. However the manual records should always be made available for the health professional's information.

6 The flowchart has also been extended to draw attention to the need to obtain the data subject's consent if a copy of any data disclosed is to be made available also to his or her general practitioner.

Action

7 RHAs, DHAs, SHAs, Family Practitioner Committees, the Dental Estimates Board and the Prescription Pricing Authority are asked to note that the Order is expected to come into effect on 11 November 1987 and to implement the provisions of this circular. This circular should be brought to the attention of health professionals, and staff with responsibilities for Data Protection matters.

From:

Health Service Division (HSlc)
Alexander Fleming House
Elephant and Castle
London SE1 6BY

Tel: 01-407 5522 Ext 6682

Further copies of this circular may be obtained from DHSS Stores, Health Publications Unit, No 2 Site, Heywood, Lancs OL10 2PZ, quoting the code and serial number appearing at the top right-hand corner.

© Crown Copyright 1987

This circular may be freely reproduced by all those to whom it is addressed.

Appendix 1

1. Children and the rights of parents

Concerning the rights of children and parents under the Data Protection Act, the Data Protection Registrar has said in Guideline 5:

'All individuals, including children, have the right of subject access. However, a child will not always be able to make his or her own request. The way in which the subject access right will work in this situation depends on the general law relating to the legal capacity of children. The law of Scotland differs in this respect from that of the rest of the United Kingdom.

'A data user in England, Wales or Northern Ireland who receives a subject access request from or on behalf of a child will need to judge whether the child understands the nature of the request.

- If the child does understand, he or she is entitled to exercise the right and the data user should reply to the child. A reply should be given to a request made on the child's behalf by a parent or guardian only if the data user is satisfied that the child has authorised the request.
- If the child does not understand, the parent or guardian is entitled to make the request on behalf of the child and to receive the reply. Parents or guardians should only make such a request in the interests of the child, not in their own interests.

'In Scotland individuals under the age of 18 are, for legal purposes, either 'pupils' or 'minors'. Until the age of minority is reached (12 years for a girl and 14 years for a boy) the child is a pupil. From that age until he or she reaches 18 the child is a minor.

- For a pupil the subject access right will be exercised by the person entitled under Scots law to act as the 'tutor' of the child – this will usually be the parent.
- Minors will be entitled to exercise the right for themselves. The data user is not required to obtain the consent of the parent or other 'curator' of the minor. A request by a minor's parent or curator should only be complied with if there is evidence that the minor has authorised the request.'

2. Policy guidance

'Data users and health authorities are reminded that the Data Protection Act is about providing access to information, not withholding it. The data user needs to be satisfied that the child understands the nature of the request; but in England and Wales this requirement may be satisfied on an interview if the application is handled personally, or by the certificate of an adult in the case of a postal application. And even with a postal application, a certificate is not essential if there is other information in the data user's possession that the child has sufficient understanding.

'In circumstances where a parent is applying on behalf of a child the data user should seek a declaration from the parent that the child either lacks capacity or has authorised the parent to make application on his or her behalf.

'The data user should accept the validity of this declaration unless there is information in his possession that the child *has* capacity (eg where a child is recorded as having given consent to a disclosure). Data users should seek the advice of the appropriate health professional to advise on whether it is known that the child in fact lacks capacity or if there are reasons to believe that the child would not wish the information to be disclosed. In these circumstances the data user should make further enquiries of the parent or child as appropriate.

'It is important not to confuse the issue of validity of subject access requests by or on behalf of children, with the separate issue of applying the modified access to personal health information provisions of the Data Protection Act.'

Note. In applying this guidance 'parent' means the person who in law is undertaking the duties and has the associated rights which are normally vested in a natural parent.

[Appendix 2 amends HC(87)14]

Data Protection Act 1984: Modified Access to Personal Health Information (HC(89)29)

DEPARTMENT OF HEALTH: HEALTH SERVICES MANAGEMENT CIRCULAR

To:

Regional Health Authorities
District Health Authorities
Special Health Authorities for the London
   Postgraduate Teaching Hospitals   } for action
Family Practitioner Committees
Dental Estimates Board
Prescription Pricing Authority

Mental Health Act Commission
Community Health Councils   } for information

November 1989

The guidance in this circular will be cancelled and deleted from the current communication index on 31 October 1994 unless notified separately.

Summary

This circular:

a. Confirms the advice in circulars HC(87)14 and HC(87)26/HC(FP)(87)9 which predated the coming into force of the Data Protection (Subject Access Modification) (Health) Order 1987 on 11 November 1987;

b. Clarifies the position of health professionals under the Data Protection Act;

c. Gives further advice on applications by children;

d. Advises further on the parental rights of access.

Action

Authorities should ensure that the contents of this circular are made known to all health professionals and to officers with responsibility for data protection matters and that revised procedures for dealing with applications by children are implemented.

From:

Health Service Division (HS1C)
Elleen House 80–94 Newington Causeway
Elephant and Castle
London SE1 6YX

Tel 01-972 2000 Ext 22729

Further copies of this circular may be obtained from DHSS Stores, Health Publications Unit, No 2 Site, Heywood, Lancs OL10 2PZ quoting the serial number appearing at the top right-hand corner.

© Crown Copyright 1989

This circular may be freely produced by all those to whom it is addressed.

Appendix

Subject Access Modification Order

1 Authorities will recall that circulars HC(87)14 and HC(87)26/HC(FP)-(87)9 gave advice on the terms of an Order which was to be laid before Parliament. The Data Protection (Subject Access Modification) (Health) Order 1987 – SI 1987/1903 – came into effect on 11 November 1987 as did a similar Order relating to social work data, the Data Protection (Subject Access Modification) (Social Work) Order 1987 – SI 1987/1904.

The position of health professionals under the Order

2 The Schedule to SI 1987/1903 lists those who are defined as health professionals for the purpose of the Order. The data user must consult the most appropriate health professional to decide whether to withhold access. In the hospital environment and community health service, in the majority of cases this will be the doctor or dentist carrying overall clinical responsibility for the patient. This practitioner should seek the advice of other health professionals who have had a significant input into the patient's care.

3 There will also be circumstances in which doctors have not been involved. It will then be appropriate for the data user to contact one of the other health professionals listed in the schedule to the Order. It is for the data user to decide who is the most appropriate health professional. In respect of work in the community, for example, the most appropriate professional is likely to be the nurse.

Applications by children

[Para 4 amends HC(87)26]

5 It is not a requirement of the Act that application forms should be used. Where standard application forms are used, data users are asked to ensure that these contain provision for a certificate on the following lines:

'**Note**. In the case of a person under the age of 18, a responsible adult should certify, where appropriate, that the child understands the nature of the application.'

[I, (name)................................. of, (address)................................

....

certify that the applicant understands the nature of this application.

(Signed)..................................... (date).......................................]

Access by parents

6 The term 'parent' is not defined in the 1984 Act. However in law 'parent' normally means the person undertaking the duties and who has the associated rights which are normally vested in a natural parent. Thus in considering whether access should be allowed to an adult in respect of a child's personal health information, account should be taken of the relationship between the adult and the child, whether the adult is the natural parent or if there has been a legal adoption or if the child has been made a ward of court.

7 Where a child lacks capacity to exercise his rights to access his own personal health information, a parent or legal guardian has the power to exercise that right on the child's behalf providing the parent or legal guardian considers it necessary to have access to the data for the purpose of carrying out the duty to take care of the child. Health authorities should assume, unless there are grounds to suggest the contrary, that a parent or legal guardian making a request on behalf of a dependent child who lacks capacity is acting in that child's best interests and access should be allowed. As in the case of adult persons, requests for health information of children will need to be viewed by the appropriate health professional.

As the data user, the health authority will have to decide in any particular circumstances whether or not to comply with the request made. Any refusal to supply the data requested may be subject to legal challenge.

What the Data Protection Act does

8 Where personal data are held on computer the Act requires that appropriate security measures shall be taken against unauthorised access to, or alteration, disclosure, or destruction of personal data and against accidental loss or destruction of personal data. The Data Protection Registrar has amplified this and has advised that the prime responsibility for creating and putting into practice a security policy must rest with the computer user; that personal data can only be accessed, altered, disclosed or destroyed by authorised people and that those people only act within the scope of their authority.

9 Where there are arrangements for joint working with the social services or other organisations and there are joint records, who is the 'data user' for these records and in responding to a request for access is a matter of fact depending upon the details of the arrangements in each case. The Data Protection Registrar's Guideline No 2 gives guidance on who is the data user and the advice of the authority's lawyer should be sought, where necessary.

Access to Health Records Act 1990

1990 CHAPTER 23

An Act to establish a right of access to health records by the individuals to whom they relate and other persons; to provide for the correction of inaccurate health records and for the avoidance of certain contractual obligations; and for connected purposes.

[13th July 1990]

Be it enacted by the Queen's most Excellent Majesty, by and with the advice and consent of the Lords Spiritual and Temporal, and Commons, in this present Parliament assembled, and by the authority of the same, as follows: –

Preliminary

'Health record' and related expressions

1 – (1) In this Act 'health record' means a record which –

(a) consists of information relating to the physical or mental health of an individual who can be identified from that information, or from that and other information in the possession of the holder of the record; and

(b) has been made by or on behalf of a health professional in connection with the care of that individual;

but does not include any record which consists of information of which the individual is, or but for any exemption would be, entitled to be supplied with a copy under section 21 of the Data Protection Act 1984 (right of access to personal data). [1984 c. 35.]

(2) In this Act 'holder', in relation to a health record, means –

(a) in the case of a record made by, or by a health professional employed by, a general practitioner –

(i) the patient's general practitioner, that is to say, the general practitioner on whose list the patient is included; or

(ii) where the patient has no general practitioner, the Family Practitioner Committee or Health Board on whose medical list the patient's most recent general practitioner was included;

(b) in the case of a record made by a health professional for purposes connected with the provision of health services by a health service body, the health service body by which or on whose behalf the record is held;

(c) in any other case, the health professional by whom or on whose behalf the record is held.

(3) In this Act 'patient', in relation to a health record, means the individual in connection with whose care the record has been made.

Health professionals

2 – (1) In this Act 'health professional' means any of the following, namely –

(a) a registered medical practitioner;

(b) a registered dentist;

(c) a registered optician;

(d) a registered pharmaceutical chemist;

(e) a registered nurse, midwife or health visitor;

(f) a registered chiropodist, dietitian, occupational therapist, orthoptist or physiotherapist;

(g) a clinical psychologist, child psychotherapist or speech therapist;

(h) an art or music therapist employed by a health service body; and

(i) a scientist employed by such a body as head of a department.

(2) Subsection (1)(a) above shall be deemed to include any person who is provisionally registered under section 15 or 21 of the Medical Act 1983 and is engaged in such employment as is mentioned in subsection (3) of that section. [1983 c. 54.]

(3) If, after the passing of this Act, an order is made under section 10 of the Professions Supplementary to Medicine Act 1960, the Secretary of State may by order make such consequential amendments of subsection (1)(f) above as may appear to him to be necessary or expedient. [1960 c. 66.]

(4) The provisions of this Act shall apply in relation to health professionals in the public service of the Crown as they apply in relation to other health professionals.

Main provisions

Right of access to health records

3 – (1) An application for access to a health record, or to any part of a health record, may be made to the holder of the record by any of the following, namely –

(a) the patient;

(b) a person authorised in writing to make the application on the patient's behalf;

(c) where the record is held in England and Wales and the patient is a child, a person having parental responsibility for the patient;

(d) where the record is held in Scotland and the patient is a pupil, a parent or guardian of the patient;

(e) where the patient is incapable of managing his own affairs, any person appointed by a court to manage those affairs; and

(f) where the patient has died, the patient's personal representative and any person who may have a claim arising out of the patient's death.

(2) Subject to section 4 below, where an application is made under subsection (1) above the holder shall, within the requisite period, give access to the record, or the part of a record, to which the application relates –

(a) in the case of a record, by allowing the applicant to inspect the record or, where section 5 below applies, an extract setting out so much of the record as is not excluded by that section;

(b) in the case of a part of a record, by allowing the applicant to inspect an extract setting out that part or, where that section applies, so much of that part as is not so excluded; or

(c) in either case, if the applicant so requires, by supplying him with a copy of the record or extract.

(3) Where any information contained in a record or extract which is so allowed to be inspected, or a copy of which is so supplied, is expressed in terms which are not intelligible without explanation, an explanation of those terms shall be provided with the record or extract, or supplied with the copy.

(4) No fee shall be required for giving access under subsection (2) above other than the following, namely –

(a) where access is given to a record, or part of a record, none of which was made after the beginning of the period of 40 days immediately preceding the date of the application, a fee not exceeding the maximum prescribed under section 21 of the Data Protection Act 1984 [1984 c. 35.]; and

(b) where a copy of a record or extract is supplied to the applicant, a fee not exceeding the cost of making the copy and (where applicable) the cost of posting it to him.

(5) For the purposes of subsection (2) above the requisite period is –

(a) where the application relates to a record, or part of a record, none of which was made before the beginning of the period of

40 days immediately preceding the date of the application, the period of 21 days beginning with that date;

(b) in any other case, the period of 40 days beginning with that date.

(6) Where –

(a) an application under subsection (1) above does not contain sufficient information to enable the holder of the record to identify the patient or, in the case of an application made otherwise than by the patient, to satisfy himself that the applicant is entitled to make the application; and

(b) within the period of 14 days beginning with the date of the application, the holder of the record requests the applicant to furnish him with such further information as he may reasonably require for that purpose,

subsection (5) above shall have effect as if for any reference to that date there were substituted a reference to the date on which that further information is so furnished.

Cases where right of access may be wholly excluded

4 – (1) Where an application is made under subsection (1)(a) or (b) of section 3 above and –

(a) in the case of a record held in England and Wales, the patient is a child; or

(b) in the case of a record held in Scotland, the patient is a pupil,

access shall not be given under subsection (2) of that section unless the holder of the record is satisfied that the patient is capable of understanding the nature of the application.

(2) Where an application is made under section (1)(c) or (d) of section 3 above, access shall not be given under subsection (2) of that section unless the holder of the record is satisfied either –

(a) that the patient has consented to the making of the application; or

(b) that the patient is incapable of understanding the nature of the application and the giving of access would be in his best interests.

(3) Where an application is made under subsection (1)(f) of section 3 above, access shall not be given under subsection (2) of that section if the record includes a note, made at the patient's request, that he did not wish access to be given on such an application.

Cases where right of access may be partially excluded

5 – (1) Access shall not be given under section 3(2) above to any part of a health record –

    (a) which, in the opinion of the holder of the record, would disclose –

        (i) information likely to cause serious harm to the physical or mental health of the patient or of any other individual; or

        (ii) information relating to or provided by an individual, other than the patient, who could be identified from that information; or

    (b) which was made before the commencement of this Act.

(2) Subsection (1)(a)(ii) above shall not apply –

    (a) where the individual concerned has consented to the application; or

    (b) where that individual is a health professional who has been involved in the care of the patient;

and subsection (1)(b) above shall not apply where and to the extent that, in the opinion of the holder of the record, the giving of access is necessary in order to make intelligible any part of the record to which access is required to be given under section 3(2) above.

(3) Where an application is made under subsection (1)(c), (d), (e) or (f) of section 3 above; access shall not be given under subsection (2) of that section to any part of the record which, in the opinion of the holder of the record, would disclose –

    (a) information provided by the patient in the expectation that it would not be disclosed to the applicant; or

    (b) information obtained as a result of any examination or investigation to which the patient consented in the expectation that the information would not be so disclosed.

(4) Where an application is made under subsection (1)(f) of section 3 above, access shall not be given under subsection (2) of that section to any part of the record which, in the opinion of the holder of the record, would disclose information which is not relevant to any claim which may arise out of the patient's death.

(5) The Secretary of State may by regulations provide that, in such circumstances as may be prescribed by the regulations, access shall not be given under section 3(2) above to any part of a health record which satisfies such conditions as may be so prescribed.

Correction of inaccurate health records

6 – (1) Where a person considers that any information contained in a health record, or any part of a health record, to which he has been given access under section 3(2) above is inaccurate, he may apply to the holder of the record for the necessary correction to be made.

(2) On an application under subsection (1) above, the holder of the record shall –

(a) if he is satisfied that the information is inaccurate, make the necessary correction;

(b) if he is not so satisfied, make in the part of the record in which the information is contained a note of the matters in respect of which the information is considered by the applicant to be inaccurate; and

(c) in either case, without requiring any fee, supply the applicant with a copy of the correction or note.

3 In this section 'inaccurate' means incorrect, misleading or incomplete.

Duty of health service bodies etc to take advice

7 – (1) A health service body or Family Practitioner Committee shall take advice from the appropriate health professional before they decide whether they are satisfied as to any matter for the purposes of this Act, or form an opinion as to any matter for those purposes.

(2) In this section 'the appropriate health professional', in relation to a health service body (other than a Health Board which is the holder of the record by virtue of section 1(2)(a) above), means –

(a) where, for purposes connected with the provision of health services by the body, one or more medical or dental practitioners are currently responsible for the clinical care of the patient, that practitioner or, as the case may be, such one of those practitioners as is the most suitable to advise the body on the matter in question;

(b) where paragraph (a) above does not apply but one or more medical or dental practitioners are available who, for purposes connected with the provision of such services by the body, have been responsible for the clinical care of the patient, that practitioner or, as the case may be, such one of those practitioners as was most recently so responsible; and

(c) where neither paragraph (a) nor paragraph (b) above applies, a health professional who has the necessary experience and qualifications to advise the body on the matter in question.

(3) In this section 'the appropriate health professional', in relation to a Family Practitioner Committee or a Health Board which is the holder of a record by virtue of section 1(2)(a) above, means –

(a) where the patient's most recent general practitioner is available, that practitioner; and

(b) where that practitioner is not available, a registered medical practitioner who has the necessary experience and qualifications to advise the Committee or Board on the matter in question.

Supplemental

Applications to the court

8 – (1) Subject to subsection (2) below, where the court is satisfied, on an application made by the person concerned within such period as may be prescribed by rules of court, that the holder of a health record has failed to comply with any requirement of this Act, the court may order the holder to comply with that requirement.

(2) The court shall not entertain an application under subsection (1) above unless it is satisfied that the applicant has taken all such steps to secure compliance with the requirement as may be prescribed by regulations made by the Secretary of State.

(3) For the purpose of subsection (2) above, the Secretary of State may by regulations require the holders of health records to make such arrangements for dealing with complaints that they have failed to comply with any requirements of this Act as may be prescribed by the regulations.

(4) For the purpose of determining any question whether an applicant is entitled to be given access under section 3(2) above to any health record, or any part of a health record, the court –

(a) may require the record or part to be made available for its own inspection; but

(b) shall not, pending determination of that question in the applicant's favour, require the record or part to be disclosed to him or his representatives whether by discovery (or, in Scotland, recovery) or otherwise.

(5) The jurisdiction conferred by this section shall be exercisable by the High Court or a county court or, in Scotland, by the Court of Session or the sheriff.

Avoidance of certain contractual terms

9 Any term or condition of a contract shall be void in so far as it purports to require an individual to supply any other person with a copy of a health record, or of an extract from a health record, to which he has been given access under section 3(2) above.

Regulations and orders

10 – (1) Regulations under this Act may make different provision for different cases or classes of cases including, in particular, different provision for different health records or classes of health records.

(2) Any power to make regulations or orders under this Act shall be exercisable by statutory instrument.

(3) Any statutory instrument containing regulations under this Act or an order under section 2(3) above shall be subject to annulment in pursuance of a resolution of either House of Parliament.

Interpretation

11 In this Act –

'application' means an application in writing and 'apply' shall be construed accordingly;

'care' includes examination, investigation, diagnosis and treatment;

'child' means an individual who has not attained the age of 16 years;

'general practitioner' means a medical practitioner who is providing general medical services in accordance with arrangements made under section 29 of the National Health Service Act 1977 or section 19 of the National Health Service (Scotland) Act 1978 [1977 c.49; 1978 c. 29.]

'Health Board' has the same meaning as in the National Health Service (Scotland) Act 1978;

'health service body' means –

(a) a health authority within the meaning of the National Health Service Act 1977;

(b) a Health Board;

(c) a State Hospital Management Committee constituted under section 91 of the Mental Health (Scotland) Act 1984 [1984 c. 36.]; or

(d) a National Health Service trust first established under section 5 of the National Health Service and Community Care Act 1990 or section 12A of the National Health Service (Scotland) Act 1978 [1990 c. 19.];

'information', in relation to a health record, includes any expression of opinion about the patient;

'make', in relation to such a record, includes compile;

'parental responsibility' has the same meaning as in the Children Act 1989 [1989 c. 41.].

Short title, commencement and extent

12 – (1) This Act may be cited as the Access to Health Records Act 1990.

(2) This Act shall come into force on 1st November 1991.

(3) This Act does not extend to Northern Ireland.

Access to Health Records Act 1990: Health Service Guidance (HSG)(91)6

Foreword

1 The Department of Health's policy has long been that, as a matter of principle, patients should be allowed to see what has been written about them. In endorsing this principle the Department has also recognised that medical records are used by doctors and other health professionals to help them in the diagnosis and treatment of patients, and that the primary purpose has been to record what is in the best interests of patients. Doctors have had to balance what is necessary to record for care and treatment purposes against the rising public expectations of greater access, and consideration of the risks which some disclosures may bring; they have exercised their professional judgement on the extent of disclosure to their patients.

2 The *Access to Health Records Act* gives patients a new right of access to their health records. In the light of this development, NHS bodies should encourage informal, voluntary arrangements whereby patients or those caring for them who, during or at the end of their treatment, ask to know what has been recorded about them, are allowed to see their records at the discretion of the health professional principally responsible for their clinical care and subject to the non-disclosure of information which might cause serious harm or identify third parties. The new Act does not prohibit such arrangements and it would be in keeping with the underlying principle of greater access to personal health information not to rely on the provisions of the Act to secure this.

Chapter 1: Background to the Act

1 The *Access to Health Records Act 1990* was a Private Member's Bill introduced by Mr Doug Henderson, MP for Newcastle-upon-Tyne North. The Act received Royal Assent on 13 July 1990 with an operative date of 1 November 1991.

2 The Act gives individuals the right of access, subject to certain exemptions, to health information about themselves recorded from 1 November 1991 other than on computer. (Health records kept on computer are already accessible to the patient by virtue of section 21 of the *Data Protection Act 1984* as modified by the *Subject Access Modification Order 1987.*)

3 The effect of the Act is essentially the same as that of the *Data Protection Act*. It therefore extends the established principles and procedures of patient access to cover all health records. Although a much greater volume of records is now covered (counterbalanced by the accelerating trend to computerised record-keeping), the Act does not introduce major changes of policy for NHS bodies or for health professionals.

Chapter 2: Outline of the Act

Note. This chapter gives an outline to the Act. As such it is not intended to be a full statement of the law. Readers who wish to be familiar with the precise statutory provisions may obtain a copy of the *Access to Health Records Act 1990* from any bookshop. The sections numbered below correspond to those in the Statutory Instrument.

Section 1
Defines the scope of the Act. It applies to records relating to the physical or mental health of an identifiable individual which have been made by a health professional in connection with care and treatment. It excludes records to which there is access under the provisions of the *Data Protection Act 1984* (ie computerised records). It defines the 'holder' of the record to whom applications for access can be made.

Section 2
Defines 'health professional' for the purposes of the Act.

Section 3
Defines those who can apply for access. In addition to the patient, they include a person authorised in writing by the patient, those acting *in loco parentis* or appointed by a court to manage the patient's affairs, personal representatives of a deceased patient and any person with a claim arising from the patient's death. It also sets out the circumstances in which a fee may be charged and the period within which access is to be given.

Section 4
Ensures that information will not be disclosed to an applicant who is not the patient against the patient's wishes or interests.

Section 5

Sets out the circumstances in which the right of access may be limited. These include circumstances in which the information might cause serious physical or mental harm to any person or disclose information about an identifiable third party without his consent. This section also provides that, even in the absence of written confirmation of his wishes, a patient's information will not be disclosed if he has provided it in the expectation that it would remain confidential.

Section 6

Allows anyone who has been allowed to see a record to ask for the correction of inaccuracies and allows the holder of the record either to correct or make a note of the alleged inaccuracy of the record.

Section 7

Imposes a duty on health service bodies to take advice from an appropriate health professional and defines the meaning of 'appropriate health professional'. (This would normally be the medical or dental practitioner responsible for the clinical care of the patient.)

Section 8

Gives an applicant a right of action in the courts if it is thought that the holder has not complied with the requirements of the Act. But the applicant must first avail himself of any arrangements to deal with complaints of non-compliance referred to in regulations. If a case gets to court, judges may inspect the health records before deciding whether the applicant should have access.

Section 9

Makes ineffective any contractual term purporting to require employees to allow employers access to their personal health information.

Section 10

Specifies the procedures for making orders or regulations under the Act.

Section 11

Defines certain terms used in the Act.

Section 12

Specifies the commencement date for the Act of 1 November 1991. The Act has only limited application to records made before that date.

Note. There is nothing in the Act which prohibits or precludes the application of any voluntary arrangements whereby health professionals exercise their existing discretion to allow their patients to see what has been entered in their health records.

Chapter 3: Definitions
What is a health record?

1 The Act defines a 'health record' in section 1(1) as meaning a record which consists of information relating to the physical or mental health of an individual who can be identified from that information, or from that and other information in the possession of the holder of the record, and which has been made by or on behalf of a health professional in connection with the care of that individual. (For the meaning of 'care', see section 11 of the Act.) It will be seen that if the record is not made in connection with the care of an individual, it does not fall within this definition. So, for example, the Act will not apply to a record about the physical or mental health of an individual which has been made in connection with the investigation of a crime. The definition applies only to records of individuals who can be identified from the information. So if information has been detached from the identity of the person to whom it relates, for example, in the context of research or medical audit, that information will not be a record to which the Act applies.

2 The Act is not confined to health records held for the purposes of the National Health Service ('the NHS'). It applies equally to the private health sector and to health professionals' private practice records. It also applies to the records, for example, of employers who hold information relating to the physical or mental health of their employees if the record has been made in connection with the care of the employee. Medical reports made for employment or insurance purposes are covered by the *Access to Medical Reports Act 1988*. There is no overlap between the two Acts.

3 Within the NHS patients registered with general medical practitioners normally have a continuous record which follows them through life and with which more than one doctor may be involved. Information recorded in the course of treatment in hospitals or by other health professionals may not have the same continuous quality. Different records may be held for different episodes of treatment in different departments or hospitals. Patients exercising their rights of access under the Act are entitled to access to the total record subject to the constraints described in Chapter 4 and not solely the episode of treatment quoted by the applicant in order to identify the relevant record. Where the patient wishes to exercise rights of access under the Act to different records, different applications may be required.

Who has the duty under the Act?

4 Obligations under the Act are, in general, placed on the holder of the record, and section 1(2) defines the 'holder'. Another of the key definitions in the Act is the definition of 'health professional' in section 2. This includes registered medical practitioners; registered dentists; registered opticians; registered pharmaceutical chemists; registered nurses, mid-wives and health visitors; registered chiropodists, dietitians, occupational therapists, orthoptists or physiotherapists; clinical psychologists, child psychotherapists or speech therapists; art or music therapists employed by a health service body; scientists employed by a health service body as heads of department. Within the NHS, the duty to give a patient access to his health record is not imposed on each of the health professionals who adds to that record. This is because in many situations, for example in a hospital, the patient's record will be compiled by many different health professionals, so that a surgeon and a physiotherapist may both add information to a patient's record. To ensure that decisions about access are made by appropriately qualified professionals, the Act provides for access to be given by the health service body (defined in section 11) after con-sultation with the appropriate health professional, normally the medical or dental practitioner who is or was responsible for the clinical care of the patient during the period to which the application refers (see section 7).

5 In relation to records made by GPs (including GDPs) or health professionals employed by them, the duty is placed on the GP on whose list the patient is, and, where there is no current GP, on the Family Practitioner Committee (now the Family Health Services Authority) on whose list the patient's most recent GP was included.

6 Where the record was made by a health professional providing health services for a district or regional health authority or NHS trust, it is that authority or NHS trust which is under the duty.

7 In any other case, the health professional by whom or on whose behalf the record is held is the person on whom the duty lies. This latter case will cover the records of most people who receive private medical services.

Who has the right of access?

8 The right of access is principally for the patient himself, and this is provided for in section 3(1) of the Act. He may also authorise another person in writing to make an application on his behalf. However, there are circumstances in which someone else has the right of access to a health record. Parents will usually have this right where the patient is a child, but there will be a need for the rights of the child to confidentiality to be balanced against the parental responsibility to ensure that only accurate and non-prejudicial information is recorded about the child. This is discussed further in Chapter 4.

9 Where a patient is incapable of managing his own affairs, it may be necessary for the person managing that person's affairs to have access.

Similarly, where the patient has died, the patient's personal representative and any person who may have a claim arising out of the patient's death have a right of access to the relevant part of the deceased's health record. Subsections (3) and (4) of section 5 prevent access to a health record by a person other than the patient where the holder is of the opinion that the patient gave the information or underwent the relevant examination or investigation in the expectation that the information would not be disclosed *to the applicant.*

Note. Where a patient is unable to manage his own affairs, the Act allows application to be made only by a person appointed by the courts. Where an adult with a learning disability is being cared for by a parent or relative who has not been appointed by the courts, the carer will not be able to exercise any right of access under the Act. Health professionals should consider the extent to which informal voluntary access (see Foreword) should be given.

Chapter 4: Providing access to health records

Applications for access

1 It is anticipated that in most cases a patient will orally request access to the records in the course of treatment, and that the health professional responsible for that episode of treatment may wish to hand the record to the patient for inspection or go through it with him. Such a request will not constitute an application under the Act.

2 In the absence of such local arrangements or if the health professional is not prepared to allow this informal access, the patient may press his right of access under the Act. The operative date under the Act is 1 November 1991. An application under the Act is required to be made in writing (see section 11). But the Act does not require that this be by the direct hand of the applicant. Staff should be ready to assist applicants in making applications. NHS bodies may wish to use a standard form for this purpose. A model form is enclosed at Appendix 1 which health authorities may wish to adapt for their own local needs.

Inspecting and copying the record

3 Although applicants may be asked for some details to help identify the relevant record, they will be entitled to see as much information as is recorded in that record, subject to the modifications set out in paragraphs 7 to 11 below.

4 Access under the Act may, in accordance with section 3(2), be afforded in one of two ways. Either the applicant may be allowed to inspect the record or the relevant part of it, or he may be entitled to inspect

an extract setting out such part of the record as he is entitled to see. In either case the applicant is entitled to be supplied with a copy of the record or extract. The applicant is entitled to an explanation of any terms which are not intelligible without explanation. The health professional should give a simple and clear explanation of the meaning of the record whether or not the applicant requests clarification.

5 A fee not exceeding that set for Data Protection Access (currently £10) may be charged when the record has not been added to in the last 40 days.

Note. The Act allows a fee of up to £10 to be charged when the record has not been added to in the last 40 days. This was intended to encourage the voluntary access arrangements referred to in the Foreword and assumed that records in such circumstances would be more readily available. A patient receiving ongoing care whose records have not been updated in the last 40 days could overcome the liability for a fee either by exercising his rights following his next booked appointment or by seeking a new appointment solely to ensure that his records are added to in a way which will allow access under the Act without a fee. Holders of records should determine their policy on fees in respect of patients receiving ongoing care who are between appointments.

Timetable for access

6 Access under the Act is to be given within 'the requisite period' which is defined in section 3(5). An application is made when the holder has enough information to enable him to deal with the application. Where the record has been made or added to within the previous 40 days, the period for giving access is 21 days from the date of the application. In other cases, the period is 40 days. Where, following an initial application, the holder of the record asks for any further information from the applicant to enable him to deal with the application, the period will run from the date the applicant provides the further information.

When may access be modified or denied?

7 The applicant will be entitled to inspect, or be supplied with a copy of, an extract rather than the whole record where section 5 applies. Section 5(1) sets out three cases where access is not to be given to the whole of a health record.

The first is the case where, in the opinion of the holder of the record, giving access would disclose information likely to cause serious harm to the physical or mental health of the patient or of any other individual.

The second is where giving access would, in the opinion of the holder of the record, disclose information relating to or provided by an individual other than the patient who could be identified from that information.

The third is where the relevant part of a health record was made before the commencement of the Act on 1 November 1991.

8 There are exceptions to the second and third rules. In relation to the second rule, access can be given where the individual who would be identified has consented to the application. Also the second rule does not apply if the individual who could be identified is a health professional involved in the care of the patient. The third rule does not apply if in the opinion of the holder of the record access needs to be given to part of the record made before 1 November 1991 if that is necessary to enable the reader to understand that part of the record to which access is being given.

9 Section 3 gives the right of access to the patient or a person authorised in writing by the patient. Section 4(1) allows the holder of the record to deny an applicant's request for access when the holder has formed the view that the patient authorising the access has not understood the meaning of the authorisation.

10 Section 4(2) covers patients who are children (ie, persons under the age of 16 years). This allows a child who, in the view of the appropriate health professional, is capable of understanding what the application is about, to prevent a person having parental responsibility from having access to the record. Where, in the view of the appropriate health professional, the child patient is not capable of understanding the nature of the application, the holder of the record is entitled to deny access if it were not felt to be in the patient's best interests.

11 Section 4(3) deals with the case where the patient has died and enables such a patient, before death, to request that a note be included in the record that he did not wish access to be given on an application.

Note. The Secretary of State has a power in section 5(5) to make regulations specifying circumstances in which access is not to be given to any part of the health record which satisfies conditions prescribed in those regulations. No exercise has yet been made of this power.

Chapter 5: Complaints of non-compliance

1 Section 8 gives an applicant a right of action in the High Court or County Court if he thinks that the holder of the record has failed to comply with any requirement of the Act.

2 An applicant may have to take a prior step before making an application to the court. Subsection (2) of section 8 gives the Secretary of State power to prescribe by regulations certain steps to secure compliance with the Act which the applicant must take before the court may entertain an application. For that purpose the Secretary of State has power to make regulations requiring a holder of health records to make arrangements for dealing with complaints that they have failed to comply with the Act.

3 Subsection (4) of section 8 gives the court a power to inspect the record or part of it itself for the purpose of determining such a question, but this would not mean that the applicant or his representatives would be entitled to see that part of the record prior to determination.

Note. At the time of preparation of this document no regulations for the review of complaints of non-compliance have been made. The Secretary of State proposes to designate the Hospital Complaints Procedures for such a purpose. NHS bodies will be notified when such regulations are made. In the absence of regulations an application to secure compliance may be made direct to the courts.

Chapter 6: Procedures for access

NHS hospitals

1 The least complicated arrangement for access to health records assumes that they have been prepared in anticipation of full access by patients subject to the health professional's discretion with regard to the non-disclosure of harmful or third party information. Such arrangements have been introduced in some parts of the NHS. Their extension to other areas, to allow patients to have information in the course of their treatment at the discretion of the health professional principally responsible for their clinical care, will minimise the administrative overheads and costs of running formal procedures.

2 In circumstances where voluntary arrangements do not exist or access has been refused, patients may wish to exercise their rights under the Act. All such applications should be processed formally and in compliance with the statutory requirements.

3 Guidelines for access to non-computerised personal health information are enclosed at Appendix 2. A flowchart summarising the procedures is at Appendix 3.

General practice records

4 As with procedures for hospitals, the most straightforward arrangements for providing access to general practice records is as part of the consultation process. Some general practitioners already provide such access on a voluntary basis and there is nothing in the Act to prohibit such arrangements.

5 In circumstances where such arrangements are not in place, patients may seek to exercise their rights under the Act to see their own records. Applications will normally be to the patient's current general practitioner or, if the patient has no current general practitioner, application may be made to the Family Health Services Authority. General practitioners and Family Health Services Authorities may wish to adapt the model form at Appendix 1 for local use.

6 The formal procedures for compliance with the Act in respect of general practice records are simpler than for applications in respect of hospital records. The general practitioner is identified by the Act as the holder of the record and there is no requirement to take advice from another appropriate health professional.

7 Where there is no current general practitioner, applications for access should be directed to the Family Health Services Authority who will be obliged to seek the advice of the patient's most recent general practitioner or, where that practitioner is not available, a registered medical practitioner who has the necessary qualifications to advise the Authority.

8 As a matter of good professional practice, general practitioners may wish to take account of views of other health professional staff employed by or attached to their practices, as well as the views of hospital based staff where this seems appropriate, eg with psychiatric records.

9 Regulations have not been made for arrangements to deal with complaints against non-compliance with the Act by general practitioners or Family Health Services Authorities. In these circumstances complainants will have a right of action direct to the High Court or County Court.

10 General practitioners and Family Health Service Authorities may wish to refer to Appendix 2 in respect of formulating their own local procedures for handling applications for access to health records.

Chapter 7: Other legislation

1 The *Data Protection Act 1984*, section 21, allows patients access to health records kept on computer, although certain information is exempt by virtue of the *Data Protection Act (Subject Access Modification) Order 1987*.

2 The *Access to Personal Files Act 1987* gives individuals a right of access to records not held on computer (so called 'manual records') held by local authorities and local social services authorities for the purposes, respectively, of their housing and social services functions.

3 The *Access to Medical Reports Act 1988* provides that an employer or insurance company cannot seek a medical report on an individual for employment or insurance purposes from the doctor responsible for that individual's care and treatment, without the individual's knowledge and consent. The individual has the right to see the report before it is passed to the employer/insurance company by the doctor commissioned to prepare the report. The individual also has the rights to request that corrections be made, and to refuse permission for the report to be passed on to the employer/insurance company.

Chapter 8: Further help and advice

1 This booklet has been prepared to guide health authorities and others in compliance with the spirit and provisions of the *Access to Health Records Act*. It is expected that readers may wish to adapt and reinforce the guidance as appropriate for local needs.

2 Health professionals may wish to take up with their professional bodies any issues of ethical or professional concern.

3 Lay staff charged with the administration and implementation of the *Access to Health Records Act* provisions may wish to know that the Association of Health Care Information and Medical Records Officers (AMRO) have developed documentation for use in the NHS. This documentation includes a request for access form (more detailed than the model form at Appendix 1), a procedure record and a control sheet for logging receipt and actions in respect of requests for access.

4 Health authorities who wish to consider adaptation of the AMRO documentation for their local purposes should direct enquiries to:

Mr N Campion
Hon. Sec
AMRO
Leefdaal
Pentre Bychan
Near Wrexham
Clwyd
North Wales

Appendix 1: Model form

Application For Access to Health Records
(Access to Health Records Act 1990)

Details of record to be accessed

Hospital/general practice: ....

Patient: Surname   ....

      Forename(s)   ....

      Date of birth   .... / .... / ....

      NHS no. if known: ....

      Hospital reference no. if known ....

Record in respect of treatment for

.... (state condition/illness if known)

about... (approximate date)

Details of applicant (if different from above)

Name: Surname   ....

      Forename(s)   ....

Declaration: I declare that the information given by me is correct to the best of my knowledge and that I am entitled to apply for access to the health record referred above under the terms of the *Access to Health Records Act 1990.*

                     * I am the patient.

                     * I have been asked to act by the patient and attach the patient's written authorisation.

                     * I am acting *in loco parentis* and the patient is under age 16 and [is incapable of understanding the request] [has consented to my making this request].

*delete as appropriate.

* I am the deceased patient's personal representative and attach confirmation of my appointment.

* I have a claim arising from the patient's death and wish to access information relevant to my claim on the grounds that:

....

....

....

....

Signed .... Date ....

Certification:

I certify that I am (Name) ....

of (address) ....

....

and that I have known the applicant for .... years as an employee/client/patient/ personal friend and have witnessed the applicant sign this form.

Signed .... Date ....

Official use only:

Fee (£10) received/not appropriate

Signed .... Date ....

Health professional advising (Name)

....

Access provided on (Date) ...... / ...... / ......

Further action: Corrections requested   Yes/No
             Applicant notified   Yes/No
                outcome
             Copies provided   Yes/No
             Copying fee (£ .....)   Yes/No
             Comments ....

....

Fee received (£ ....)

Signature .... Date ....

* delete as appropriate.

Appendix 2: Guidelines for access to hospital records in accordance with the *Access to Health Records Act 1990*

This Act gives individuals the right of access, by application in writing and subject to certain exemptions to information about themselves in manually held records in connection with their case by health professionals. The Act applies primarily to records made on or after 1 November 1991.

Administration

1 Each access application must be examined immediately to confirm its validity. If the application does not contain sufficient information to identify the record to be accessed or to confirm the right of the applicant to request access a request for further details must be issued within 14 days. (The statutory time limit for providing access commences from the date when the application has been made and the holder has all the necessary information to process the application. It is not a pre-requisite that any fee should first be paid. Receipt of an application should be logged.)

2 The application may be made by a patient, by a person authorised by the patient, by a person *in loco parentis*, by a person authorised to act on behalf of the patient, or by a deceased patient's personal representative or a person who might have a claim arising from the patient's death.

3 Further enquiries may be needed to confirm the *bona fides* of applicants other than the patient before access is given.

4 Where the applicant is not the patient, the applicant should have access to only the information which would otherwise have been made available to the patient; or which is in the best interests of the patient. Where the patient has died, disclosure would be subject to the recorded wishes of the deceased patient. If the application is in respect of a claim arising from the patient's death, access should not be given to information which is not relevant to the claim.

5 Once the necessary details have been received, the period within which a response has to be made is 40 days in respect of patients whose records have not been updated in the 40 days preceding the application. For patients whose records have been updated in the last 40 days, the Act assumes that the records will be more readily available and that the application will be simpler to process. For these applications a response within 21 days must be given.

6 Because it is easier to locate records while a patient is receiving treatment or has recently been discharged and records have been updated in the last 40 days, access should be given without a fee (other than to cover any photocopying or postage charges). In circumstances where the records were updated more than 40 days before, the Act allows that a fee *may* be charged which is not to exceed the sum prescribed under the *Data Protection Act 1984* (currently £10) and in addition to any photocopying or postage charges where applicable. [**Note:** see Chapter 4, paragraph 5.]

Consultation with health professionals

7 Where the holder of the records is a health service body defined in section 11 as a health authority within the meaning of the *National Health Service Act 1977*, a National Health Service Trust, or Family Health Services Authority, that body must take advice from the appropriate health professional about any matter on which they are to form an opinion under the Act.

8 The holder should obtain the record so that the appropriate health professional can be identified and the papers referred for his advice.

9 The appropriate health professional is the medical or dental practitioner (normally the consultant or the most recent GP) who has clinical responsibility for the particular episode of treatment to the record of which the applicant seeks to have access. This practitioner may wish to seek the views of other health professionals who have had a significant input to the patient's care. If the appropriate health professional is not available or has not had clinical responsibility for the patient, the holder should seek the advice of the health professional who seems most appropriate to advise on the application, eg another doctor or dentist, a nurse, midwife, health visitor or a clinical psychologist.

10 The appropriate health professional should advise on:
   (i)   whether access should be allowed or limited to prevent the disclosure of seriously harmful information or which might identify third party individuals;
   (ii) whether in connection with an application for access to a child's record the child is capable of understanding the nature and purpose of the application;
   (iii) whether access would be in accord with the best interests or wishes of the patient;
   Notes (a) When an applicant has a claim which may arise from the patient's death only relevant information should be disclosed.

(b) These are the only circumstances in which access may be limited or excluded. The fact that a record has not been prepared in anticipation that it might be opened to the patient is no justification for denying access under the Act.

(iv) whether access to a part of the record preceding 1 November 1991 should be allowed to make intelligible that part of the record to which access will be given under the Act;

(v) whether the applicant should be allowed to inspect the record itself or should be shown an extract setting out so much of the record as is not excluded from access. If an extract is to be shown this must be prepared by the health professional;

(vi) whether it is necessary for the health professional to be present when the record or extract is inspected (in order to provide any explanation or counselling) or if this can be supervised by a lay administrator;

(vii) whether access should be given by posting the record or extract to the applicant together with any necessary explanation.

Arrangements for disclosure

Note. The fact that information has been withheld could be as harmful to patients as the information itself. Holders are free to advise applicants the grounds on which information has been withheld but if this is thought likely to cause undue distress the holder may not wish to volunteer the fact that information has been withheld. If confronted with a direct request as to whether access has been given to the whole of the record a holder is entitled to respond that the requirements under the Act as to access have been fully complied with and may wish to refer to a summary of rights under the Act and provide the applicant with a copy of these. (See Appendix 4.) Consideration should be given to whether the applicant should be offered counselling to allay anxieties.

11 Where it is advised that an explanation or counselling is required, or where harmful information has been withheld, an appointment should be made for the applicant to inspect the record or extract with the health professional (or other health professional acting on his behalf).

12 Where the health professional advises that the access can be supervised without the attendance of a health professional, an appointment should be made for supervision by a lay administrator. In these circumstances the lay administrator must not comment or advise on the content of the record and if the applicant raises enquiries, an appointment with a health professional should be offered.

13 Following conclusion of the inspection the application form should be noted and attached to the record.

Corrections requested?

14 An applicant can apply for inaccuracies in the record to be corrected. The health professional should either make the necessary correction or make a note in the relevant part of the record of the matters alleged to be inaccurate. The applicant must be provided, without charge, with a copy of the correction or the note. Although the Act is not specific in the way in which a correction should be made, care must be taken not to simply obliterate information which may have significance for the future care and treatment of the patient or for litigation purposes. Consideration should be given to whether it is appropriate to note also any associated records.

Copies

15 The holder may charge a fee, not to exceed the costs of copying and postage where appropriate, to cover the administrative costs incurred in meeting the applicant's request for copies of the records to which he has had or would be allowed to have access.

Complaints

16 Applicants should be advised that the Act provides a right of action in the courts if the holder of the record has failed to comply with the Act. The Act also provides that the applicant must avail himself of any arrangements required under regulations by the Secretary of State for dealing with complaints of non-compliance before making an application to the courts.

17 The Secretary of State proposes to make regulations requiring NHS hospitals (directly managed units and NHS Trusts) to process complaints of non-compliance within the arrangements prescribed by the *Hospital Complaints Procedures Act 1985*. Health authorities will be notified as soon as the regulations have been made. In the interim, complaints about non-compliance can be taken direct to the courts and complainants do not have to use the hospital complaints procedures. Nevertheless complainants should be offered this facility and be advised how to contact the designated officer for complaints in the unit concerned and should be given every assistance in framing their complaint.

Disposal

18 When all administrative action has been taken the record should be returned to the appropriate location.

Appendix 3: Flowchart for access to hospital records

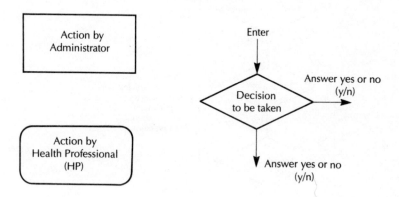

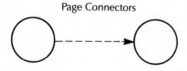

Key to Symbols Used

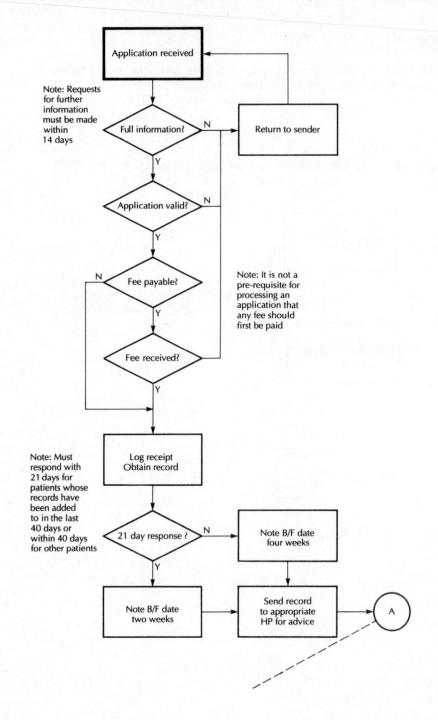

Continued on page 153

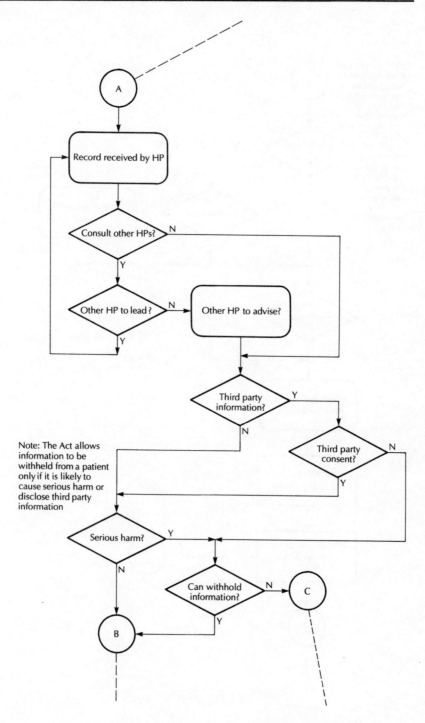

Note: The Act allows
information to be
withheld from a patient
only if it is likely to
cause serious harm or
disclose third party
information

Continued on page 154

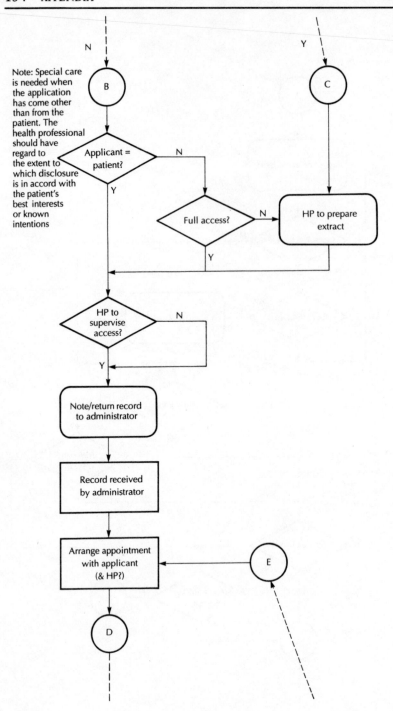

Note: Special care is needed when the application has come other than from the patient. The health professional should have regard to the extent to which disclosure is in accord with the patient's best interests or known intentions

Contd.

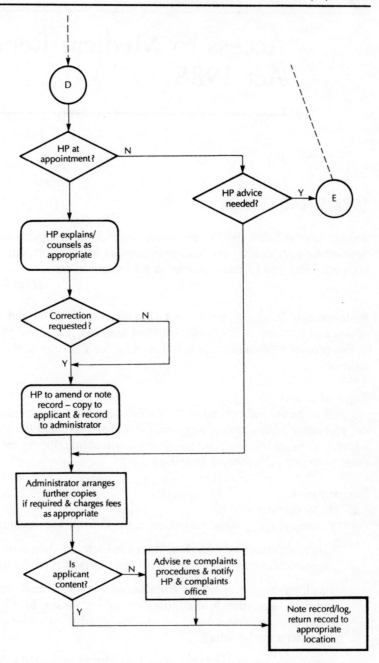

Access to Medical Reports Act 1988

1988 CHAPTER 28

An Act to establish a right of access by individuals to reports relating to themselves provided by medical practitioners for employment or insurance purposes and to make provision for related matters.

[29th July 1988]

Be it enacted by the Queen's most Excellent Majesty, by and with the advice and consent of the Lords Spiritual and Temporal, and Commons, in this present Parliament assembled, and by the authority of the same, as follows: –

Right of access
1 It shall be the right of an individual to have access, in accordance with the provisions of this Act, to any medical report relating to the individual which is to be, or has been, supplied by a medical practitioner for employment purposes or insurance purposes.

Interpretation
2 – (1) In this Act –
'the applicant' means the person referred to in section 3(1) below;

'care' includes examination, investigation or diagnosis for the purposes of, or in connection with, any form of medical treatment;

'employment purposes', in the case of any individual, means the purposes in relation to the individual of any person by whom he is or has been, or is seeking to be, employed (whether under a contract of service or otherwise);

'health professional' has the same meaning as in the Data Protection (Subject Access Modification) (Health) Order 1987 [S.I. 1987/1903.];

'insurance purposes', in the case of any individual, means the purposes in relation to the individual of any person carrying on an insurance business with whom the individual has entered into, or is seeking to enter into, a contract of insurance, and 'insurance business' and 'contract of insurance' have the same meaning as in the Insurance Companies Act 1982 [1982 c. 50.];

'medical practitioner' means a person registered under the Medical Act 1983 [1983 c. 54.];

'medical report', in the case of an individual, means a report relating to the physical or mental health of the individual prepared by a medical practitioner who is or has been responsible for the clinical care of the individual.

(2) Any reference in this Act to the supply of a medical report for employment or insurance purposes shall be construed –

(a) as a reference to the supply of such a report for employment or insurance purposes which are purposes of the person who is seeking to be supplied with it; or

(b) (in the case of a report that has already been supplied) as a reference to the supply of such a report for employment or insurance purposes which, at the time of its being supplied, were purposes of the person to whom it was supplied.

Consent to applications for medical reports for employment or insurance purposes

3 – (1) A person shall not apply to a medical practitioner for a medical report relating to any individual to be supplied to him for employment or insurance purposes unless –

(a) that person ('the applicant') has notified the individual that he proposes to make the application; and

(b) the individual has notified the applicant that he consents to the making of the application.

(2) Any notification given under subsection (1)(a) above must inform the individual of his rights to withhold his consent to the making of the application, and of the following rights under this Act, namely –

(a) the rights arising under sections 4(1) to (3) and 6(2) below with respect to access to the report before or after it is supplied;

(b) the right to withhold consent under subsection (1) of section 5 below; and

(c) the right to request the amendment of the report under subsection (2) of that section;

as well as of the effect of section 7 below.

Access to reports before they are supplied

4 – (1) An individual who gives his consent under section 3 above to the making of an application shall be entitled, when giving his consent, to state that he wishes to have access to the report to be supplied in response to the application before it is so supplied; and, if he does so, the applicant shall –

(a) notify the medical practitioner of that fact at the time when the application is made; and

(b) at the same time notify the individual of the making of the application;

and each such notification shall contain a statement of the effect of subsection (2) below.

(2) Where a medical practitioner is notified by the applicant under subsection (1) above that the individual in question wishes to have access to the report before it is supplied, the practitioner shall not supply the report unless –

(a) he has given the individual access to it and any requirements of section 5 below have been complied with; or

(b) the period of 21 days beginning with the date of the making of the application has elapsed without his having received any communication from the individual concerning arrangements for the individual to have access to it.

(3) Where a medical practitioner –

(a) receives an application for a medical report to be supplied for employment or insurance purposes without being notified by the applicant as mentioned in subsection (1) above; but

(b) before supplying the report receives a notification from the individual that he wishes to have access to the report before it is supplied;

the practitioner shall not supply the report unless –

(i) he has given the individual access to it and any requirements of section 5 below have been complied with; or

(ii) the period of 21 days beginning with the date of that notification has elapsed without his having received (either with that notification or otherwise) any communication from the individual concerning arrangements for the individual to have access to it.

(4) References in this section and section 5 below to giving an individual access to a medical report are references to –

(a) making the report or a copy of it available for his inspection; or

(b) supplying him with a copy of it;

and where a copy is supplied at the request, or otherwise with the consent, of the individual the practitioner may charge a reasonable fee to cover the costs of supplying it.

Consent to supplying of report and correction of errors

5 – (1) Where an individual has been given access to a report under section 4 above the report shall not be supplied in response to the application in question unless the individual has notified the medical practitioner that he consents to its being so supplied.

(2) The individual shall be entitled, before giving his consent under subsection (1) above, to request the medical practitioner to amend any part of the report which the individual considers to be incorrect or misleading; and, if the individual does so, the practitioner –

(a) if he is to any extent prepared to accede to the individual's request, shall amend the report accordingly;

(b) if he is to any extent not prepared to accede to it but the individual requests him to attach to the report a statement of the individual's views in respect of any part of the report which he is declining to amend, shall attach such a statement to the report.

(3) Any request made by an individual under subsection (2) above shall be made in writing.

Retention of reports

6 – (1) A copy of any medical report which a medical practitioner has supplied for employment or insurance purposes shall be retained by him for at least six months from the date on which it was supplied.

(2) A medical practitioner shall, if so requested by an individual, give the individual access to any medical report relating to him which the practitioner has supplied for employment or insurance purposes in the previous six months.

(3) The reference in subsection (2) above to giving an individual access to a medical report is a reference to –

(a) making a copy of the report available for his inspection; or

(b) supplying him with a copy of it;

and where a copy is supplied at the request, or otherwise with the consent, of the individual the practitioner may charge a reasonable fee to cover the costs of supplying it.

Exemptions

7 – (1) A medical practitioner shall not be obliged to give an individual access, in accordance with the provisions of section 4(4) or 6(3) above, to any part of a medical report whose disclosure would in the opinion of the practitioner be likely to cause serious harm to the physical or mental health of the individual or others or would indicate the intentions of the practitioner in respect of the individual.

(2) A medical practitioner shall not be obliged to give an individual access, in accordance with those provisions, to any part of a medical report whose disclosure would be likely to reveal information about another person, or to reveal the identity of another person who has supplied information to the practitioner about the individual, unless –

(a) that person has consented; or
(b) that person is a health professional who has been involved in the care of the individual and the information relates to or has been provided by the professional in that capacity.

(3) Where it appears to a medical practitioner that subsection (1) or (2) above is applicable to any part (but not the whole) of a medical report –

(a) he shall notify the individual of that fact; and
(b) references in the preceding sections of this Act to the individual being given access to the report shall be construed as references to his being given access to the remainder of it;

and other references to the report in sections 4(4), 5(2) and 6(3) above shall similarly be construed as references to the remainder of the report.

(4) Where it appears to a medical practitioner that subsection (1) or (2) above is applicable to the whole of a medical report –

(a) he shall notify the individual of that fact; but
(b) he shall not supply the report unless he is notified by the individual that the individual consents to its being supplied;

and accordingly, if he is so notified by the individual, the restrictions imposed by section 4(2) and (3) above on the supply of the report shall not have effect in relation to it.

Application to the court

8 – (1) If a court is satisfied on the application of an individual that any person, in connection with a medical report relating to that individual, has failed or is likely to fail to comply with any requirement of this Act, the court may order that person to comply with that requirement.

(2) The jurisdiction conferred by this section shall be exercisable by a county court or, in Scotland, by the sheriff.

Notifications under this Act

9 Any notification required or authorised to be given under this Act –

(a) shall be given in writing; and

(b) may be given by post.

Short title, commencement and extent

10 – (1) This Act may be cited as the Access to Medical Reports Act 1988.

(2) This Act shall come into force on 1st January 1989.

(3) Nothing in this Act applies to a medical report prepared before the coming into force of this Act.

(4) This Act does not extend to Northern Ireland.

Access and Litigation

4

Supply of Information about Hospital Patients in the Context of Civil Legal Proceedings (HC(82)16)

DEPARTMENT OF HEALTH AND SOCIAL SECURITY: HEALTH SERVICE MANAGEMENT CIRCULAR

To:

Regional Health Authorities
District Health Authorities
Special Health Authorities for
   London Postgraduate Teaching Hospitals
Boards of Governors

} for action

Family Practitioner Committees
Community Health Councils

} for information

September 1982

Summary

This Circular draws attention to recent legislation concerning the powers of the High Court to order disclosure of documents before and in proceedings for personal injury or death and sets it in the context of existing guidance on voluntary disclosure of information about hospital patients contemplating or engaged in civil legal proceedings.

Existing guidance and practice

1 Guidance on the voluntary release of information about patients contemplating or engaged in civil legal proceedings is contained in HM(59)88. Paragraphs 3 and 4 (the texts of which are reproduced at

Annex A) advise on the action to be taken by health authorities when a request for case notes or information from them is received from the patient concerned or his representative. This advice remains applicable, in particular that authorities should not stand on their strict rights in these circumstances and that the doctor concerned must always be consulted where medical matters are in any way involved.

2 It has since become a widely accepted practice for disclosure in these circumstances to be made to the applicant's medical adviser. This practice is commended as a means of ensuring that case notes are correctly interpreted for the applicant's benefit.

Powers of High Court to order disclosure in advance of proceedings

3 In addition to the inherent power to order disclosure between parties to proceedings which have been commenced the High Court has for some years had powers to order disclosure of relevant documents where the applicant and the person ordered to make disclosure are both likely to be parties to proceedings in cases of personal injury or death (and to order disclosure to a party to such proceedings which have commenced from someone who is not a party to them). Such powers were first conferred in the Administration of Justice Act 1970. A decision of the House of Lords in 1978 in a Northern Ireland case (McIvor v Southern Health and Social Services Board) established that under the Act, if the court did make an order, the documents would have to be made available to the applicant and that there was no power to restrict disclosure, as had earlier been the practice, to a medical or other adviser of the applicant. HN(78)95, which is cancelled by this Circular, drew the attention of authorities to this decision.

4 Since then, there have been further changes in the law and the relevant powers of the High Court, as amended, are now contained in sections 33(2) and 34(1) and (2) of the Supreme Court Act 1981. The text of these sections is reproduced in Annex B, together with that of section 35 which contains supplementary provisions. Under the new law, which came into operation on 1 January 1982, the court has power to order production to the applicant or, on such conditions as may be specified in the order, to –

  (a) the applicant's legal advisers; or
  (b) the applicant's legal advisers and any medical or other professional adviser of the applicant; or
  (c) if the applicant has no legal adviser, to any medical or other professional adviser of the applicant.

Requests for information from patients

5 In considering requests from patients or their authorised representatives* for disclosure of case notes or information from them in connection with actual or possible litigation, authorities should continue to observe the spirit of HM(59)88. In cases of doubt account should be taken of the powers of the High Court to order disclosure in advance of proceedings. It would not be appropriate for health authorities to adopt a more stringent test than would be likely to be applied by the court when considering an application under section 33(2) or 34(2) of that Act since this could have the effect of forcing the applicant to resort to court action when there was no real doubt as to the outcome. Authorities are reminded that for the purpose of an order under section 33(2) of the Act the applicant would not need to convince the court of the merits of his claim against the authority, but he would, under the Rules of the Supreme Court, be required to state the grounds on which he was likely to be a party to subsequent proceedings.

Requests from third parties for information about patients

6 Where a request (as opposed to a subpoena or court order) for information is received not from the patient himself or his authorised representative but from some other party engaged in or contemplating legal proceedings with him, the information requested should not be supplied without the written consent of the patient concerned and of the doctor concerned where medical matters are in any way involved. This replaces the advice in paragraph 5 of HM(59)88 which is withdrawn.

Action on receiving an order or subpoena

7 Any health authority officer (for example, a hospital medical records officer) who is served with a court order or subpoena for the production of case notes or the giving of evidence based on them should immediately notify the District Administrator. The District Administrator should notify the doctor concerned (normally the consultant in charge of the case, or his successor) and should consider whether the authority's legal advisers and any other members of staff concerned should be informed. While there should be no delay in acting on the order, in cases of doubt the authority's

---

*'Authorised representative' in this context means anyone who the authority is satisfied is acting on behalf of the patient with the patient's consent in the actual or proposed litigation or, where the patient is deceased or incapable of giving consent, is legally entitled to act on behalf of him or his estate.

and the doctor's legal advisers may need to advise on whether an appeal should be entered against it. In complying with an order for the production of documents care should be taken to ensure that the documents are made available only to the person or persons to whom the court has ordered the production, and that any conditions specified in the order are observed.

Fees for supplying information

8 The circumstances in which a member of the medical staff of the hospital may charge a fee for supplying information are covered in the Schedules of Category I and II work set out in the Handbook of Terms and Conditions of Service for Hospital Medical and Dental Staff. Paragraph 6 of HM(59)88 is withdrawn.

Cancellation of earlier guidance

9 The following are cancelled:

HM(59)88, paragraphs 5 and 6 (paragraph 8 was cancelled by HM(61)110); HN(78)95; HN(80)32.

Action

10 Health authorities are asked to bring the contents of this Circular to the attention of all staff who may be involved with orders or requests for disclosure of information about patients.

From:

Children's Division D, Alexander Fleming House, Elephant and Castle, London SE1 6BY

Annex A (HC(82)16): Supply of information about hospital patients engaged in legal proceedings (extract from HM(59)88)

3 Where a request for records or reports is made on what are manifestly insubstantial grounds, the hospital cannot be expected to grant it, but where information is being sought in pursuance of a claim of prima facie substance against the Board or Committee or a member of their staff or both, the decision is more difficult and each request must be examined on its own merits, in the light of legal advice, and of course in consultation with any member of their medical or dental staff directly concerned in the outcome of the claim (in this connection see HM(54)32). The production of case notes and similar documents is not obligatory before the stage of discovery in the actual proceedings is reached,* but the Minister does not feel that boards and committees, especially as they are public authorities, would either wish or be well advised to maintain their strict rights in this connection except for some good reason bearing on the defence to the particular claim or on the ground that the request is made without substantial justification.

4 Where the information is required in a matter which has nothing to do with the hospital or any member of its staff, for example in litigation between the patient and a third party, hospital authorities should be prepared to help by providing, as far as possible, the information asked for subject always to the consent of the patient.** Sometimes the information sought may be entirely unrelated to medical matters – for example the date of the patient's admission or discharge; whether he was a private patient and signed the appropriate form of undertaking; and if so, the amount paid by way of hospital charges. Such information may properly be given by the Secretary of the board or committee, without reference to the medical staff. But in all cases – and they will undoubtedly be the majority – where medical matters are in any way involved (for example where information is wanted about the diagnosis made on admission, details of treatment, conditions on discharge, or prognosis) the doctor or dentist who was in charge of the patient's treatment at the hospital, or his successor, should be consulted. It is self-evident that this must be done when a medical or dental report is being asked for. But the principle is equally important when the request is only for extracts from the case notes, since it is necessary for the doctor or dentist to ensure that any extracts which are made are not misleading, and also that their disclosure to the patient cannot in any way be harmful medically to him – it would no doubt often be undesirable to let the patient himself have so detailed a report or such full extracts from the medical records as it would be proper to give to his general practitioner. This decision is one which can be made only by a professionally qualified person. At the same time it is imperative that no material information which can in any way be relevant to the matter should be withheld in such a way as to convey a wrong picture.

Annex B (HC(82)16): Supreme Court Act 1981

33 – (2) On the application, in accordance with rules of court, a person who appears to the High Court to be likely to be a party to subsequent

---

* There is now an exception to this, namely where a court order is made under the Supreme Court Act 1981 (see paragraph 4 of the main body of this Circular).

** Where the request for information is not from the patient himself or his authorised representative see paragraph 6 of the main body of the Circular.

proceedings in that court in which a claim in respect of personal injuries to a person, or in respect of a person's death, is likely to be made, the High Court shall, in such circumstances as may be specified in the rules, have power to order a person who appears to the court to be likely to be a party to the proceedings and to be likely to have or to have had in his possession, custody or power any documents which are relevant to an issue arising or likely to arise out of that claim –

   (a)   to disclose whether those documents are in his possession, custody or power; and

   (b)   to produce such of those documents as are in his possession, custody or power to the applicant or, on such conditions as may be specified in the order –

      (i)   to the applicant's legal advisers; or

      (ii)   to the applicant's legal advisers and any medical or other professional adviser of the applicant; or

      (iii) if the applicant has no legal adviser, to any medical or other professional adviser of the applicant.

34 – (1) This section applies to any proceedings in the High Court in which a claim is made in respect of personal injuries to a person, or in respect of a person's death.

(2) On the application, in accordance with rules of court, of a party to any proceedings to which this section applies, the High Court shall, in such circumstances as may be specified in the rules, have power to order a person who is not a party to the proceedings and who appears to the court to be likely to have in his possession, custody or power any documents which are relevant to an issue arising out of the said claim –

   (a)   to disclose whether those documents are in his possession, custody or power; and

   (b)   to produce such of those documents as are in his possession, custody or power to the applicant or, on such conditions as may be specified in the order –

      (i)   to the applicant's legal advisers; or

      (ii)   to the applicant's legal advisers and any medical or other professional adviser of the applicant; or

      (iii) if the applicant has no legal adviser, to any medical or other professional adviser of the applicant.

(3) On the application, in accordance with rules of court, of a party of any proceedings to which this section applies, the High Court shall, in such circumstances as may be specified in the rules, have power to make an order providing for any one or more of the following matters, that is to say –

   (a)   the inspection, photographing, preservation, custody and detention of property which is not the property of, or in the possession of, any party to the proceedings but which is the subject-matter of the proceedings or as to which any question arises in the proceedings;

(b) the taking of samples of any such property as is mentioned in paragraph (a) and the carrying out of any experiment on or with any such property.

(4) The preceding provisions of this section are without prejudice to the exercise by the High Court of any power to make orders which is exercisable apart from those provisions.

35 – (1) The High Court shall not make an order under section 33 or 34 if it considers that compliance with the order, if made, would be likely to be injurious to the public interest.

(2) Rules of court may make provision as to the circumstances in which an order under section 33 or 34 can be made; and any rules making such provision may include such incidental, supplementary and consequential provisions as the rule-making authority may consider necessary or expedient.

(3) Without prejudice to the generality of subsection (2), rules of court shall be made for the purpose of ensuring that the costs of and incidental to proceedings for an order under section 33(2) or 34 incurred by the person against whom the order is sought shall be awarded to that person unless the court otherwise directs.

(4) Sections 33(2) and 34 and this section bind the Crown; and section 33(1) binds the Crown so far as it relates to property as to which it appears to the court that it may become the subject-matter of subsequent proceedings involving a claim in respect of a person's death.

In this subsection references to the Crown do not include references to Her Majesty in Her private capacity or to Her Majesty in right of Her Duchy of Lancaster or to the Duke of Cornwall.

(5) In sections 33 and 34 and this section –

'property' includes any land, chattel or other corporeal property of any description;

'personal injuries' includes any disease and any impairment of a person's physical or mental condition.

Index

Note. Page references in **bold** refer to statutes and circulars reproduced in the Appendix.